Foreword

T5-DHC-878

There is an ancient notion that the art and the science of medicine must coexist in tension—the former being humanistic while the latter mechanistic. Although this has been exposed as fallacious since the time of Hippocrates, the misconception has proven durable. For example we recall not-so-fondly a recent past when psychology, psychiatry, and social work were relegated to the back burner of clinical research in oncology. Heady with technical improvements in the management of cancer, many in our community haughtily endorsed a biocentrism that placed little emphasis on emotional, social, and spiritual distress. "Why worry about the patient's psyche," they said, "when all we need to do is to shrink the cancer and everything else will get better on its own?" Others, often less mainstream but no less vocal, championed a science-phobic "love conquers all" approach. They eschewed intellectual rigor in favor of intuitive compassion in the pursuit of a holistic cancer medicine. While seeming to disagree, advocates of the two views actually shared an acceptance of a body-mind polarity, divided only by which side was most important. Fortunately for all of us, the insight, clarity of thought, and perseverance of the pioneers of psychosocial oncology (represented so well in the authorship of this book) have enlightened us. As illustrated herein we now have tools that permit us to reflect on the mind as well as the body with both rigor and compassion. But to continue moving forward we must apply and extend these advances in common practice, which is what this book is all about. Using it well will help us better evaluate and care for the whole patient, who has always needed and has always deserved both our most scientific art and our most artful science.

Larry Norton, MD
Deputy Physician-in-Chief for Breast Cancer Programs
Memorial Sloan-Kettering Cancer Center

Note to readers: The pharmacological dosage information in this handbook has been carefully reviewed. However, the drug manufacturers' current indications, dosage information and drug interaction warnings should be consulted prior to prescribing any drug listed in this work. Some forms listed may not be readily available and other forms may become available.

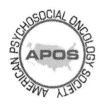

ISBN-10 0-9785319-0-6
ISBN-13 978-0-9785319-0-4

Single copies of this book may be ordered by using the form in the back of the book or by contacting:

American Psychosocial Oncology Society
2365 Hunters Way
Charlottesville, VA 22911, USA

Tel: +1.434.293.5350
Fax: +1.434.977.1856
E-mail: info@apos-society.org

Published through IPOS Press. IPOS Press is a publishing entity of the International Psycho-Oncology Society (IPOS).

Contents

Continued, next page

Contents, continued

Contributing Authors

Sarah S. Auchincloss, MD
Consultant in Psychiatry
Memorial Sloan-Kettering Cancer Center
New York, New York

Walter F. Baile, MD
Professor and Chief, Psychiatry
University of Texas MD Anderson
Cancer Center
Houston, Texas

Stewart B. Fleishman, MD
Director, Cancer Supportive Services
Continuum Cancer Center of New York
Beth Israel & St Lukes Roosevelt
New York, New York

Mitch Golant, PhD
Vice-President, Research and
Development
The Wellness Community
Los Angeles, California

Donna B. Greenberg, MD
Associate Professor, Psychiatry
Harvard Medical School;
Director, Psychiatric Oncology Service
Massachusetts General Hospital
Cancer Center
Boston, Massachusetts

Rev. George F. Handzo
The Health Care Chaplaincy
New York, New York

Jimmie C. Holland, MD
Attending Psychiatrist
Memorial Sloan-Kettering Cancer Center
New York, New York

Mary K. Hughes, MS, RN, CNS, CT
Clinical Nurse Specialist
University of Texas MD Anderson
Cancer Center
Houston, Texas

Ann A. Jakubowski, MD, PhD
Memorial Sloan-Kettering Cancer Center
New York, New York

Kenneth L. Kirsh, PhD
Assistant Professor, Pharmacy Practice
and Science
University of Kentucky
Lexington, Kentucky

David W. Kissane, MD
Chairman, Department of Psychiatry and
Behavioral Sciences
Memorial Sloan-Kettering Cancer Center
New York, New York

Jon A. Levenson, MD
Associate Clinical Professor of Psychiatry
Columbia University, College of
Physicians and Surgeons;
Attending Psychiatrist
Presbyterian Hospital
New York, New York

Continued, next page

Contributing Authors, continued

Matthew J. Loscalzo, MSW
Associate Clinical Professor of
Medicine, Hematology-Oncology;
Co-Director, Palliative Care;
Director of Patient and Family Support
Rebecca and John Moores UCSD
Cancer Center
La Jolla, California

Mary Jane Massie, MD
Attending Psychiatrist
Memorial Sloan-Kettering Cancer Center
New York, New York

Anna C. Muriel, MD, MPH
Massachusetts General Hospital;
Instructor in Psychiatry
Harvard Medical School
Boston, Massachusetts

Steven D. Passik, PhD
Associate Attending Psychologist
Memorial Sloan-Kettering Cancer Center
New York, New York

William F. Pirl, MD
Director, Cancer-related Fatigue Clinic
Massachusetts General Hospital
Boston, Massachusetts

Paula K. Rauch, MD
Chief, Child Psychiatry
Consultation Service
Massachusetts General Hospital;
Assistant Professor of Psychiatry
Harvard Medical School
Boston, Massachusetts

Inga Reznik, PhD
Clinical Psychologist
Memorial Sloan-Kettering Cancer Center
New York, New York

Andrew J. Roth, MD
Associate Attending Psychiatrist
Memorial Sloan-Kettering Cancer
Center;
Associate Professor
Weill Medical College of Cornell
University
New York, New York

Alan D. Valentine, MD
University of Texas MD Anderson
Cancer Center
Houston, Texas

Margo W. Walsh, PhD
Psycho-Oncologist
Hematology Oncology Northwest
Tacoma, Washington

1 Purpose and Overview

This book is directed primarily to you—the oncologists and nurses who are working in today's busy clinical oncology settings. You are often joined on the "front line" by social workers who, with you, constitute the first line of defense for recognizing the distress of patients and their families that accompanies the diagnoses and treatment of cancer. This small handbook aims to provide the essential facts needed to help you to identify rapidly and diagnose the common psychiatric disorders; to know the optimal medication management for them; the common psychosocial problems of patients and families; the role of spiritual and religious issues in coping; and, to offer a simple tool and algorithm for referring the patient, when needed, for evaluation by a mental health professional. We believe this handbook provides useful information to all members of the clinical team who treat patients. We expect that the guidelines will help in teaching medical, nursing and social work students. Mental health professionals working in the psychological, psychiatric and psychosocial aspects of care – those who back up the primary oncology team in this area—will find it a good overview for themselves and an introduction for students.

The goal of this handbook is to improve the recognition and optimal management of distress in patients with cancer in the context of their total oncologic care, and to provide you with a short "curbside consult"—in book or PDA form—just as you would ask for from a mental health colleague in the hallway or clinic. The early diagnosis and referral of patients who are distressed will lead to better satisfaction with care; fewer serious psychiatric problems that cause disruptions in clinic and hospital settings; improved doctor-patient communication; trust and respect will be increased. Most importantly, patients' ability to adhere to their oncologic treatment is enhanced when they are freed of troublesome symptoms of distress. The added benefit is less stress for the oncology team.

The book addresses the assumption that there can be no well defined clearcut standards or guidelines for the care of the psyche of patients with cancer. The National Comprehensive Cancer Network (NCCN) addressed this basic issue in 1997. It established a multidisciplinary panel, using the model that NCCN has used to develop clinical practice guidelines for treatment of major tumors and common symptoms of pain, nausea and vomiting, and fatigue. The panel, comprised of oncologists, oncology nurses, social workers, psychologists, psychiatrists, clergy and patients—all agreed that mental function is a critical component as patients fight cancer, cope with treatments and deal with the uncertainty of survival. They also recognized the stigma attached to mental issues, and the fact that there was at that time, no definition of optimal state-of-the art psychiatric and psychosocial care of patients with cancer, and hence no standard of care to which clinics and hospitals could be held accountable.

As a result of the panel's deliberations, the NCCN Distress Management Guidelines[1] were written in the same NCCN format and algorithms familiar to oncologists. (Available at www.nccn.org with links to Supportive and End of Life care). The guidelines articulate common serious and treatable psychiatric syndromes, offer a differential diagnosis for distress, and consider the psychological, social, and spiritual component of symptoms like fatigue and pain. The chapters in the handbook present these common psychiatric disorders and psychosocial and spiritual problems, using the NCCN Distress Management Guidelines and the same format.

Figure 1.1   NCCN Distress Management Guidelines DIS-5 - Expected Distress Symptoms[1]

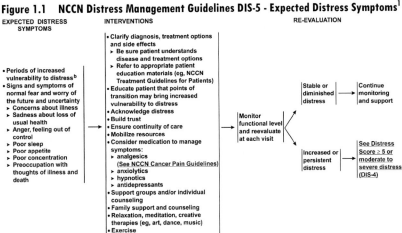

© National Comprehensive Cancer Network, May 2005

The panel addressed the core issue of stigma: patients are reluctant to reveal emotional problems, and doctors who are busy may not ask. The "don't ask, don't tell" policy led the panel to recommend the use of the word "distress" which is more acceptable to patients and staff than "psychiatric" and "psychosocial." Since it is normal and expected to experience distress with a cancer diagnosis, this term is readily understood. These "expected" distress symptoms are outlined on Figure 1.1 as well as the range of interventions available to the oncologist, nurse and social worker.

First and foremost, communication reduces distress, so assure a level of communication that clarifies the diagnosis and treatment options, allows time for questions, and puts the patient at ease. Acknowledge that cancer treatment is a difficult experience and that distress is expected. If patients feel that they can express feelings of distress to the staff, they are somewhat relieved, and the process builds trust. Patients need to feel the primary team's commitment and their genuine concern for the patient's total care. The clinical judgement of the patient's distress, whether it is appropriate to the context, a serious and treatable psychiatric problem, or a barrier to medical treatment is not straightforward. It may challenge the time resources and expertise of the oncology team.

Since clinically significant distress is overlooked in many patients, the panel recommends screening for distress level using a simple tool, the Distress Thermometer (Figure 1.2),[2,3] similar to the 0 - 10 rating scale used to ask patients about their level of pain. This one-response measure of overall distress captures some of the qualities of lengthier depression screening tools, but only takes a moment to complete.

The Problem List accompanies the Thermometer, asking the patient to indicate the causes of their distress, as to whether they are practical, family, emotional, spiritual or physical. The panel recommends that the single sheet of paper be given to the patient in the waiting room (Figure 1.2). The patients places a mark on the scale answering: "How distressed have you been this past week, including today?" As with the pain-rating scale,

Figure 1.2   NCCN Distress Management Guidelines DIS-A - Distress Thermometer[2,3]

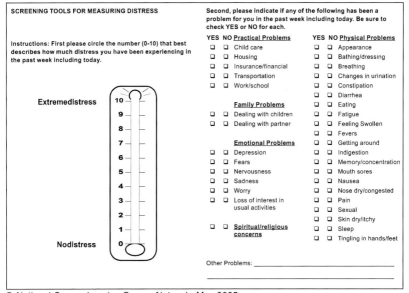

© National Comprehensive Cancer Network, May 2005

scores of 5 or more indicate a significant level of distress that should be evaluated further. This score has been validated against instruments which are longer, and it is a valid tool for an initial rough screen of distress with the cut-off score around 4 - 5. When screening tools for psychological distress have been applied in outpatient clinics, approximately one third of patients are found to be experiencing significant levels of distress, greater in those who have tumors with a poorer prognosis.[4] The screening tool calls attention to the distressed patient and allows the conversation about distress to begin. The single question can be asked verbally as well as using a paper-and-pencil approach.

Since the oncology nurse is present at all visits, she is the likely person to look at the Thermometer and Problem List and may ask any clarifying questions in the treatment room. Social workers are often not immediately available in busy clinics to perform this function. If the patient's level of distress is mild (below 4 - 5), the primary oncology team will manage the normal fears, worries and uncertainties (Figure 1.3). If the patient marks 5 or greater, this is an indication of a level of distress that should be evaluated further and the score serves as the algorithm for referral to a mental health professional, social worker or clergy.

Figure 1.3 shows an overview of the evaluation and triage process from the NCCN Distress Management Guidelines,[5] with the score of 4 - 5 or more serving to differentiate moderate to severe distress from mild that the team will manage. Psychiatrists and psychologists, social workers, and clergy will then manage the patients, using the NCCN Guidelines for the DSM IV psychiatric diagnoses for mental health professionals,

Figure 1.3   NCCN Distress Management Guidelines DIS-4 - Evaluation and Treatment[5]

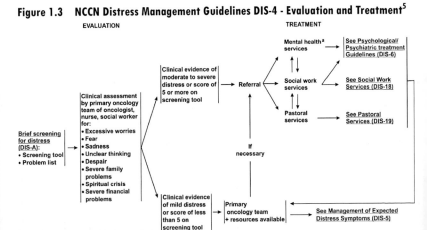

© *National Comprehensive Cancer Network, May 2005*

guidelines for social work in the practical and psychosocial areas, and guidelines for the management of the problems which are commonly seen by clergy and chaplain (e.g. grief, concerns about afterlife, feelings of abandonment by God). An assumption of these guidelines is that mental health providers can work with each other and with the oncology team, see the same patients, and refer to each other. The guidelines presume that referrals are placed to trained staff who will meet the standards of their discipline.

References:

1. Expected Distress Symptoms (DIS-5). Reproduced with permission from the *NCCN 1.2005 Distress Management, The Complete Library of NCCN Clinical Practice Guidelines in Oncology [CD-Rom]*. Jenkintown, Pennsylvania: ©National Comprehensive Cancer Network, May 2005. To view the most recent and complete version of the guidelines, go online to www.nccn.org.*

2. Distress Thermometer (DIS-A). Reproduced with permission from the *NCCN 1.2005 Distress Management, The Complete Library of NCCN Clinical Practice Guidelines in Oncology [CD-Rom]*. Jenkintown, Pennsylvania: ©National Comprehensive Cancer Network, May 2005. To view the most recent and complete version of the guidelines, go online to www.nccn.org.*

3. Jacobsen PB, Donovan KA, Trask, PC, Fleishman, SB, Zabora, J, Baker F, et al. (2004). Screening for psychologic distress in ambulatory cancer patients: A multicenter evaluation of the distress thermometer. *Cancer, 103*, 1494-1502.

4. Zabora J, BrintzenhofeSzoc K, Curbow, B, Hooker C & Piantadosi S (2001). The prevalence of psychological distress by cancer site. *Psycho-Oncology, 10*, 19-28.

5. Overview of Evaluation and Treatment Process (DIS-4). Reproduced with permission from the *NCCN 1.2005 Distress Management, The Complete Library of NCCN Clinical Practice Guidelines in Oncology [CD-Rom]*. Jenkintown, Pennsylvania: ©National Comprehensive Cancer Network, May 2005. To view the most recent and complete version of the guidelines, go online to www.nccn.org.*

2 Screening Instruments

Introduction

Many instruments have been developed to assess psychosocial distress and its subtypes in cancer patients. While you may not employ them often in clinical care, they do help in identifying the presence and severity of a particular symptom. This chapter provides a guide to these instruments. The chapter is organized according the NCCN Distress algorithm, starting with a single-item tool to assess general psychosocial distress rapidly in the waiting room (The Distress Thermometer, Figure 2.1) and then focusing on more specific areas of distress as the clinical evaluation proceeds.

General Distress

Distress Thermometer - Figure 2.1[1]

The distress thermometer is a 0-10 scale that asks patients to rate their distress. Scores of 4 or above should have further evaluation. The tool also contains a list of possible problems that patients can check to guide your evaluation of the distress and its appropriate treatment. These problems include practical problems, family problems (cf. Chapter 8), emotional problems (cf. Chapter 6), spiritual/religious concerns (cf. Chapter 8), and physical problems (cf. Chapter 7). If a patient checks, "yes," to an item under "Emotional Problems," you could consider giving them the Hospital Anxiety and Depression Scale (HADS, Figure 2.2) and/or the Zung Depression Rating Scale (ZDRS, Figure 2.3) for more specific assessment. If a patient checks, "yes," to an item under Spiritual/religious Concerns, you might consider evaluating this further by taking a spiritual history with the FICA questions (Figure 2.8) under the heading of "Spirituality." If a patient checks, "yes," to problems with "memory/concentration" under "Physical Problems," consider further assessment with the Mini Mental Status Examination (MMSE, Figure 2.4).

Some forms of distress may not be readily identified by the Distress Thermometer such as substance abuse, dementia, and delirium. Based on the patient's history and clinical presentation, other assessments should be done for further evaluation. For substance abuse, consider the CAGE questions (Figure 2.7) described under the heading of "Substance Abuse." If there is concern about possible dementia, tests under the heading, "Cognition," the MMSE (Figure 2.4) and the Clock Drawing Test (Figure 2.5), should be considered. If there is concern about delirium, the tests under the "Cognition" heading, including the Memorial Delirium Assessment Scale (MDAS, Figure 2.6) should be considered.

Figure 2.1   NCCN Distress Management Guideline DIS-A - Distress Thermometer[1]

SCREENING TOOLS FOR MEASURING DISTRESS

Instructions: First please circle the number (0-10) that best describes how much distress you have been experiencing in the past week including today.

Extremedistress 10

9

8

7

6

5

4

3

2

1

Nodistress 0

Second, please indicate if any of the following has been a problem for you in the past week including today. Be sure to check YES or NO for each.

YES NO Practical Problems
☐ ☐ Child care
☐ ☐ Housing
☐ ☐ Insurance/financial
☐ ☐ Transportation
☐ ☐ Work/school

Family Problems
☐ ☐ Dealing with children
☐ ☐ Dealing with partner

Emotional Problems
☐ ☐ Depression
☐ ☐ Fears
☐ ☐ Nervousness
☐ ☐ Sadness
☐ ☐ Worry
☐ ☐ Loss of interest in usual activities

☐ ☐ **Spiritual/religious concerns**

YES NO Physical Problems
☐ ☐ Appearance
☐ ☐ Bathing/dressing
☐ ☐ Breathing
☐ ☐ Changes in urination
☐ ☐ Constipation
☐ ☐ Diarrhea
☐ ☐ Eating
☐ ☐ Fatigue
☐ ☐ Feeling Swollen
☐ ☐ Fevers
☐ ☐ Getting around
☐ ☐ Indigestion
☐ ☐ Memory/concentration
☐ ☐ Mouth sores
☐ ☐ Nausea
☐ ☐ Nose dry/congested
☐ ☐ Pain
☐ ☐ Sexual
☐ ☐ Skin dry/itchy
☐ ☐ Sleep
☐ ☐ Tingling in hands/feet

Other Problems: _____
_____

© *National Comprehensive Cancer Network, May 2005*

Emotional Problems

Hospital Anxiety and Depression Scale (HADS) - Figure 2.2[2]

The HADS is a 14-item self-report instrument that assesses both anxiety and depressive symptoms. The instrument was designed for medically ill patients and does not include physical symptoms. The HADS contains seven items that assess anxiety and seven items that assess depression. A total score is derived from all fourteen items with sub-scales for anxiety and depression. It has been validated in patients with cancer and may be the most widely used instrument to assess depressive symptoms in cancer patients. Scores on the HADS do not diagnose anxiety and mood disorders; they measure the severity of symptoms which suggest the likeliness that a patient may have a disorder. A total score of 15 or greater or a score of 8 or greater on a sub-scale suggests that a patient may have a anxiety or mood disorder. However, in psychosocial research, the cut-off scores for the HADS can vary and some believe that higher scores are necessary to increase the specificity of the instrument. (Cf. Chapter 6, Mood Disorders.)

Figure 2.2[2]   *HADS*

Please read each item and CIRCLE the answer that comes closest to how you have been feeling, on the average, IN THE PAST WEEK. Don't spend too much time on your answers: Your immediate reaction to each item will probably be more accurate than a long thought-out response.

1. **I feel tense or "wound up":**
   a. Most of the time
   b. A lot of the time
   c. From time to time
   d. Not at all

2. **I still enjoy the things I used to enjoy:**
   a. Definitely as much
   b. Not quite so much
   c. Only a little
   d. Hardly at all

3. **I get a sort of frightened feeling as if something awful is about to happen:**
   a. Very definitely and quite badly
   b. Yes, but not too badly
   c. A little, but it doesn't worry me
   d. Not at all

4. **I can laugh and see the funny side of things:**
   a. As much as I always could
   b. Not quite so much now
   c. Definitely not so much now
   d. Not at all

5. **Worrying thoughts go through my mind:**
   a. A great deal of the time
   b. A lot of the time
   c. From time too time but not too often
   d. Only occasionally

6. **I feel cheerful:**
   a. Not at all
   b. Not often
   c. Sometimes
   d. Most of the time

7. **I can sit at ease and feel relaxed:**
   a. Definitely
   b. Usually
   c. Not often
   d. Not at all

8. **I feel as if I am slowed down:**
   a. Nearly all the time
   b. Very often
   c. Sometimes
   d. Not at all

9. **I get a sort of frightened feeling like "butterflies" in my stomach:**
   a. Not at all
   b. Occasionally
   c. Quite often
   d. Very often

10. **I have lost interest in my appearance:**
    a. Definitely
    b. I don't take as much care as I should
    c. I may not take quite as much care
    d. I take just as much care as ever

11. **I feel restless as if I have to be on the move:**
    a. Very much indeed
    b. Quite a lot
    c. Not very much
    d. Not at all

12. **I look forward with enjoyment to things:**
    a. As much as I ever did
    b. Rather less than I used to
    c. Definitely less than I used to
    d. Hardly at all

13. **I get sudden feelings of panic:**
    a. Very often indeed
    b. Quite often
    c. Not very often
    d. Not at all

14. **I can enjoy a good book or radio or TV program:**
    a. Often
    b. Sometimes
    c. Not often
    d. Very seldom

Zung Depression Rating Scale (ZDRS) - Figure 2.3[3]

The ZDRS is a 20-item self-report instrument that measures the level and severity of depressive symptoms. Scores range from 20 to 80 and scores above 48 are suggestive of at least mild depression. A short version (11-items) has been used in cancer patients that does not include the nine items that refer to somatic symptoms. This scale has been used successfully in an algorithm for depression treatment in an oncology clinic.[4,5]

Figure 2.3[3]   <u>Zung Self-Rating Depression Scale</u>

Make check mark in appropriate column ☑	A little of the time	Some of the time	Good part of the time	Most of the time
1. I feel downhearted and blue.				
2. Morning is when I feel the best.				
3. I have crying spells or feel like it.				
4. I have trouble sleeping at night.				
5. I eat as much as I used to.				
6. I still enjoy sex.				
7. I notice that I am losing weight.				
8. I have trouble with constipation.				
9. My heart beats faster than usual.				
10. I get tired for no reason.				
11. My mind is as clear as it used to be.				
12. I find it easy to do the things I used to.				
13. I am restless and can't keep still.				
14. I feel hopeful about the future				
15. I am more irritable than usual.				
16. I find it easy to make decisions.				
17. I feel that I am useful and needed.				
18. My life is pretty full.				
19. I feel that others would be better off if I were dead.				
20. I still enjoy the things I used to.				

Cognition

Mini Mental Status Examination (MMSE) - Figure 2.4, Parts 1 - 3[6]

The MMSE is a 14-item clinician-administered instrument to assess cognition, regardless of cause. It contains items on orientation, attention, recall, visual-spatial construction, and language abilities. Scores of 24 or less suggest severe impairment. Further neuropsychological assessment is often needed for dementia, particularly assessments that include tests of frontal lobe functioning. The MMSE can be used serially to follow patients at risk for developing cognitive impairment or patients who have had alterations in their cognition, particularly by delirium. (Cf. Chapter 6, Cognitive Disorders.)

Figure 2.4, Part 1[6]

INSTRUCTIONS FOR ADMINISTRATION OF
MINI MENTAL STATUS EXAMINATION

ORIENTATION

1. Ask for the date. Then ask specifically for parts omitted. i.e., "Can you also tell me what season it is?" One point for each correct.
2. Ask in turn, "Can you tell me the name of this place?", town, county, etc. One point for each correct.

REGISTRATION

Tell the person you are going to test their memory. Then say the names of three unrelated objects, clearly and slowly, about one second for each. After you have said all three, ask him to repeat them. This first repetition determines his score (0-3) but keep saying them until he can repeat all three, up to six trials. If the subject does not eventually learn all three, recall cannot be meaningfully tested.

ATTENTION AND CALCULATION

Ask the subject to begin with 100 and count backwards by 7. Stop after five subtractions. Score the total number of correct answers.

If the subject cannot or will not perform this task, ask him to spell the word "world" backwards. The score is the number of letters in correct order, i.e., dlrow = 5 points, dlorw = 3 points.

RECALL

Ask the patient if he can recall the three words you previously asked him to remember. One point for each correctly recalled.

LANGUAGE

Naming: Show the subject a wristwatch and ask her what it is.
Repeat with a pencil. One point for each named correctly.

Repetition: Ask the patient to repeat the sentence after you. Allow only one trial.

3 Stage Command: give the verbal instructions, then present the subject a sheet of paper. One point for each part of the command that is correctly executed.

Reading: Have the subject read the phrase "CLOSE YOUR EYES". The letters should be large and dark enough for the subject to read. Ask him to "Read the sentence and do what it says." Score correctly only if they read the phrase and close their eyes.

Writing: Give the subject a blank piece of paper and ask her write a sentence for you. Do not dictate a sentence, it is to be written by the subject spontaneously. To score correctly, it must contain a subject and verb and be sensible. It should be a complete thought. Correct grammar and punctuation are NOT necessary.

Copying: On a piece of paper, draw intersecting pentagons, each side about one inch and ask him to copy it exactly as it is. To score correctly, all ten angles must be present AND two must intersect. Tremor and rotation are ignored.

Estimate the subject's level of sensorium along a continuum, from alert to coma.

TOTAL SCORE POSSIBLE = 30
23 OR LESS: HIGH LIKELIHOOD OF DEMENTIA
25-30: NORMAL AGING OR BORDERLINE DEMENTIA

Figure 2.4, Part 3[6]

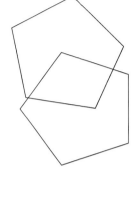

Close your eyes.

Figure 2.4, Part 2[6]

MINI MENTAL STATUS EXAM

PATEINT'S NAME: _____

Date: _____ Client's Highest Level of Education: _____

Maximum Score	Score	
		ORIENTATION
5	( )	What is the (year) (season) (date) (day) (month)?
5	( )	where are we: (state) (county) (town) (hospital) (floor)?
		REGISTRATION
3	( )	Name 3 objects: One syllable words, 1 seco'nd to say each. Then ask the patient all 3 after you have said them.
		Give 1 point for each correct answer. Then repeat them until he learns all 3.
		Count trials and record. Trials _____
		ATTENTION AND CALCULATION
5	( )	Serial 7's. 1 point for each correct. Stop after 5 answers. Alternatively spell "world" backwards. 100 − 93 − 86 − 79 − 72 − 65 − 58
		RECALL
3	( )	Ask for 3 objects repeated above. Give 1 point for each correct.
		LANGUAGE
9	( )	Name a pencil, and watch (2 points)
	( )	Repeat the following: "No ifs, and or buts." (1 point)
	( )	Follow a 3-stage command: "Take this paper in your right hand, fold it in half, and put it on the floor." (3 points)
	( )	Read and obey the following: "Close your eyes" (1 point)
	( )	Write a sentence. (1 point)
	( )	Copy design. (1 point)

_____ Total Score

Assess level of consciousness along a continuum.   (Alert) (Drowsy) (Stupor) (Coma)

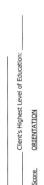

Clock Drawing Test - Figure 2.5[7,8,9]

The Clock Drawing Test is a pen-and-paper test that assesses several cognitive abilities. It is a good adjuvant test of executive functioning when given with the MMSE (pp. 9 - 11).[7] Patients are asked to draw a clock on a piece of paper, putting the numbers on the face, and making the hands on the clock designate a specific time, such as ten minutes before two. This task tests patients' ability to follow complex commands, sequence and plan their actions, and visual-spatial ability. The drawn clock can be objectively scored by a validated scoring system. There are two scoring systems, each of which has reasonable sensitivity and specificity in identifying cognitive dysfunction.[8,9] In the Sunderland, et al., method, scores of 6 or more are considered normal. (Cf. Chapter 6, Cognitive Disorders.)

Figure 2.5

Please draw the numbers on the circle to make it look like a clock. Then please draw the hands of the clock to read 10 past 11.

Watson et al. Scoring Method[8]

1. Divide the circle into 4 equal quadrants by drawing one line through the center of the circle and the number 12 (or a mark that best corresponds to the 12) and a second line perpendicular to and bisecting the first.
2. Count the number of digits in each quadrant in the clockwise direction, beginning with the digit corresponding to the number 12. Each digit is counted only once. If a digit falls on one of the reference lines, it is included in the quadrant that is clockwise to the line. A total of 3 digits in a quadrant is considered to be correct.
3. For any error in the number of digits in the first, second or third quadrants assign a score of 1. For any error in the number of digits in the fourth quadrant assign a score of 4.
4. Normal range of score is 0-3. Abnormal (demented) range of score is 4-7.

Sunderland et al. Scoring Method[9]

Score

10-6 Drawing of clock face with circle and number is generally intact.

10   Hands are in correct position.

9   Slight errors in placement of the hands.

8   More noticeable errors in the placement of hour and minute hands.

7   Placement of hands is significantly off course.

6   Inappropriate use of clock hands (i.e. use of digital display or circling of numbers despite repeated instructions).

5-1 Drawing of clock face with circle and numbers is *not* intact.

5   Crowding of numbers at one end of the clock or reversal of numbers. Hands may still be present in some fashion.

4   Further distortion of number sequence. Integrity of clock face is now gone (i.e. numbers missing or placed at outside of the boundaries of the clock face).

3   Numbers and clock face no longer obviously connected in the drawing. Hands are not present.

2   Drawing reveals some evidence of instructions being received but only a vague representation of a clock.

1   Either no attempt or an uninterpretable effort is made.

Memorial Delirium Assessment Scale (MDAS) (1) - Figure 2.6

The Memorial Delirium Assessment Scale (MDAS) is a ten-item clinician-administered assessment that evaluates the areas of cognition most sensitive to impairment with delirium: arousal, level of consciousness, memory, attention, orientation, disturbances in thinking, and psychomotor activity. Scores range from 0-30. A score of 13 or above suggests delirium. This scale, used serially, monitors changes in function. (Cf. Chapter 6, Cognitive Disorders.)

Figure 2.6[10]

Memorial Delirium Assessment Scale

Instructions: Rate the severity of the following symptoms of delirium based on current interaction with subject or assessment of his/her behavior or experience over past several hours (as indicated in each time).

ITEM 1 - REDUCED LEVEL OF CONSCIOUSNESS (AWARENESS):
Rate the patient's current awareness of and interaction with the environment (interviewer, other people/objects in the room; for example, ask patients to describe their surroundings).

- ☐ 0: none (patient spontaneously fully aware of environment and interacts appropriately)
- ☐ 1: mild (patient is unaware of some elements in the environment or is not spontaneously interacting appropriately with the interviewer; becomes fully aware and appropriately interactive when prodded strongly; interview is prolonged but not seriously disrupted)
- ☐ 2: moderate (patient is unaware of some or all elements in the environment or is not spontaneously interacting with the interviewer; becomes incompletely aware and inappropriately interactive when prodded strongly; interview is prolonged but not seriously disrupted)
- ☐ 3: severe (patient is unaware of all elements in the environment with no spontaneous interaction or awareness of the interviewer so that the interview is difficult to impossible, even with maximal prodding)

ITEM 2 - DISORIENTATION: Rate current state by asking the following 10 orientation items: date, month, day, year, season, floor, name of hospital, city, state, and country.

- ☐ 0: none (patient knows 9-10 items)
- ☐ 1: mild (patient knows 7-8 items)
- ☐ 2: moderate (patient knows 5-6 items)
- ☐ 3: severe (patient knows no more than 4 items)

Continued through page 16

ITEM 3 - SHORT-TERM MEMORY IMPAIRMENT: Rate current state by using repetition and delayed recall of 3 words [patient must immediately repeat and recall words 5 minutes later after an intervening task. Use alternate sets of 3 words for successive evaluations (e.g., apple, table, tomorrow; sky, cigar, justice)].

- ☐ 0: none (all 3 words repeated and recalled)
- ☐ 1: mild (all 3 repeated; patient fails to recall 1)
- ☐ 2: moderate (all 3 repeated; patient fails to recall 2-3)
- ☐ 3: severe (patient fails to repeat 1 or more words)

ITEM 4 - IMPAIRED DIGIT SPAN: Rate current performance by asking subjects to repeat first 3, 4, then 5 digits forward and then 3, then 4 backward; continue to the next step only if patient succeeds at the previous one.

- ☐ 0: none (patient can do at least 5 numbers forward, 4 backward)
- ☐ 1: mild (patient can do at least 5 numbers forward, 3 backward)
- ☐ 2: moderate (patient can do 4-5 numbers forward, cannot do 3 backward)
- ☐ 3: severe (patient can do no more than 3 numbers forward)

ITEM 5 - REDUCED ABILITY TO MAINTAIN AND SHIFT ATTENTION: As indicated during the interview by questions needing to be rephrased and/or repeated because patient's attention wanders, patient loses track, patient is distracted by outside stimuli or overabsorbed in task.

- ☐ 0: none (none of the above; patient maintains and shifts attention normally)
- ☐ 1: mild (above attentional problems occur once or twice without prolonging the interview)
- ☐ 2: moderate (above attentional problems occur often, prolonging the interview without seriously disrupting it)
- ☐ 3: severe (above attentional problems occur constantly, disrupting and making the interview difficult to impossible)

ITEM 6 - DISORGANIZED THINKING: As indicated during the interview by rambling, irrelevant or incoherent speech, or by tangential, circumstantial, or faulty reasoning. Ask patient a somewhat complex question (e.g., "Describe your current medical condition.").

- ☐ 0: none (patient's speech is coherent and goal-directed)
- ☐ 1: mild (patient's speech is slightly difficult to follow; responses to questions are slightly off target but not so much as to prolong the interview)
- ☐ 2: moderate (disorganized thoughts or speech are clearly present, such that interview is prolonged but not disrupted)
- ☐ 3: severe (examination is very difficult or impossible due to disorganized thinking or speech)

Continued through page 16

ITEM 7 - PERCEPTUAL DISTURBANCE: Misperceptions, illusions, hallucinations inferred from inappropriate behavior during the interview or admitted by the subject, as well as those elicited from nurse/family/chart accounts of the past several hours or of the time since last examination:

☐ 0: none (no misperceptions, illusions, or hallucinations)

☐ 1: mild (misperceptions or illusions related to sleep, fleeting hallucinations on 1-2 occasions without inappropriate behavior)

☐ 2: moderate (hallucinations or frequent illusions on several occasions with minimal inappropriate behavior that does not disrupt the interview)

☐ 3: severe (frequent or intense illusions or hallucinations with persistent inappropriate behavior that disrupts the interview or interferes with medical care)

ITEM 8 - DELUSIONS: Rate delusions inferred from inappropriate behavior exhibited during the interview or admitted by the patient, as well as delusions elicited from nurse/family/chart accounts of the past several hours or of the time since the previous examination.

☐ 0: none (no evidence of misinterpretations or delusions)

☐ 1: mild (misinterpretation or suspiciousness without clear delusional ideas or inappropriate behavior)

☐ 2: moderate (delusions admitted by the patient or evidenced by his/her behavior that do not or only marginally disrupt the interview or interfere with medical care)

☐ 3: severe (persistent and/or intense delusions resulting in inappropriate behavior, disrupting the interview or seriously interfering with medical care)

ITEM 9 - DECREASED OR INCREASED PSYCHOMOTOR ACTIVITY: Rate activity over past several hours, as well as activity during interview, by circling (a) hypoactive, (b) hyperactive, or (c) elements of both present.

☐ 0: none (normal psychomotor activity)

a b c ☐ 1: mild (Hypoactivity is barely noticeable, expressed as slightly slowing movement. Hyperactivity is barely noticeable or appears as simple restlessness.)

a b c ☐ 2: moderate (Hypoactivity is undeniable, with marked reductions in the number of movements or marked slowness of movement; subject rarely spontaneously moves or speaks. Hyperactivity is undeniable; subject moves almost constantly; in both cases, exam is prolonged as a consequence.)

a b c ☐ 3: severe (Hypoactivity is severe; patient does not move or speak without prodding or is catatonic. Hyperactivity is severe; patient is constantly moving, overreacts to stimuli, requires surveillance and/or restraint; getting through the exam is difficult or impossible.)

Continued through page 16

ITEM 10 - SLEEP-WAKE CYCLE DISTURBANCE (DISORDER OR AROUSAL): Rate patient's ability to either sleep or stay awake at the appropriate times. Utilize direct observation during the interview, as well as reports from nurses, family, patient, or charts describing sleep-wake cycle disturbance over the past several hours or since last examination. Use observations of the previous night for morning evaluations only.

- ☐ 0: none (at night, sleeps well; during the day, has no trouble staying awake)
- ☐ 1: mild (mild deviation from appropriate sleepfulness and wakefulness states; at night, difficulty falling asleep or transient night awakenings, needs medication to sleep well; during the day, reports periods of drowsiness or, during the interview, is drowsy but can easily fully awaken him/herself)
- ☐ 2: moderate (moderate deviations from appropriate sleepfulness and wakefulness states; at night, repeated and prolonged night awakening; during the day, reports of frequent and prolonged napping or, during the interview, can only be roused to complete wakefulness by strong stimuli)
- ☐ 3: severe (severe deviations from appropriate sleepfulness and wakefulness states; at night, sleeplessness; during the day, patient spends most of the time sleeping or, during the interview, cannot be roused to full wakefulness by any stimuli)

SUBSTANCE ABUSE

CAGE Questions - Figure 2.7[11]

Substance use is evaluated to assess substance abuse or dependence. The CAGE questions help guide the assessment of alcohol abuse. CAGE is an acronym for the four questions below. A "yes" answer to at least two of these questions suggests alcohol abuse or dependence. (Cf. Chapter 6, Substance Abuse.)

Figure 2.7[11]

1. Have you ever felt the need to **C**ut down?
   Yes   No

2. Do you get **A**nnoyed when other people are critical of your drinking?
   Yes   No

3. Do you feel **G**uilty about using?
   Yes   No

4. Have you ever needed an **E**ye-opener in the morning?
   Yes   No

SPIRITUALITY

8. FICA Questions - Figure 2.8[12]

Spirituality is an important part of many people's lives and provides a sense of connectedness and comfort during times of illness and distress. Cancer often precipitates a spiritual crisis as a person searches for meaning in their life and illness. Spirituality is evaluated by questions around four main themes to guide your history taking and give you a better sense of the patient's dependence on spirituality in coping with illness. They are not scored and focus on strengths. The four themes can be remembered using the acronym, FICA. (Cf. Chapter 8, Spiritual/Religious Communication.)

Figure 2.8   FICA Questions (Revised by the Author Subsequent to Initial Publication)[12]

Faith & Belief: "Do you consider yourself spiritual or religious?" or "Do you have spiritual beliefs that help you cope with stress or difficult times?" If the patient responds "no," the physician might ask, "What gives your life meaning?" Sometime patients respond with answers such as family, career, or nature.

Importance: "What importance does your faith or belief have in your life? Have your beliefs influenced how you take care of yourself in this illness? What role do your beliefs play in regaining your health?"

Community: "Are you a part of a spiritual or religious community? Is this of support to you and how? Is there a group of people you really love or who are important to you?" Communities, such as churches, temples, mosques, or a group of like-minded friends, can serve as strong support systems for some patients.

Address/**A**ction in Care: The physician and other health care providers can think about what needs to be done with the information the patient shared—referral to chaplain, other spiritual care provider, or other resource.

© 2000 by Christina M. Puchalski, MD, FACP[12]

References

1.   Screening Tools for Measuring Distress. Reproduced with permission from the *NCCN 1.2005 Distress Management, The Complete Library of NCCN Clinical Practice Guidelines in Oncology [CD-Rom]*. Jenkintown, Pennsylvania: ©National Comprehensive Cancer Network, May 2005. To view the most recent and complete version of the guidelines, go online to www.nccn.org.*

2.   Zigmond AS & Snaith RP (1983). The hospital anxiety and depression scale. *Acta Anaesthesiologica Scandinavica*, 67, 361-370.

3.   Zung WWK (1965). A self-rating depression scale. *Archives of General Psychiatry*, 12, 63-70.

4. Passik SD, Kirsh KL, Donaghy KB, Theobald DE, Lundberg JC, Holtsclaw E, et al. (2001). An attempt to employ the Zung Self-Rating Depression Scale as a "lab test" to trigger follow-up in ambulatory oncology clinics – criterion validity and detection. Journal of Pain and Symptom Management, 21, 273-281.

5. Passik SD, Lundberg JC, Rosenfeld B, Kirsh KL, Donaghy K, Theobald D, et al. (2000). Factor analysis of the Zung Self-Rating Depression Scale in a large ambulatory oncology sample. Psychosomatics, 41, 121-127.

6. Folstein MF, Folstein SE & McHugh PR (1975). "Mini-mental state." A practical method for grading the cognitive state of patients for the clinician. Journal of Psychiatric Research, 12, 189-198.

7. Juby A, Tench S & Baker V (2002). The value of clock drawing in identifying executive cognitive dysfunction in people with a normal Mini-Mental State Examination score. Canadian Medical Association Journal, 167, 859-864.

8. Watson YI, Arfken CL & Birge SJ (1993). Clock completion: An objective screening test for dementia. Journal of the American Geriatrics Society, 41, 1235-1240.

9. Sunderland T, Hill JL, Mellow AM, Lawlor BA, Gundersheimer J, Newhouse PA, et al. (1989). Clock drawing in Alzheimer's disease: A novel measure of dementia severity. Journal of the American Geriatrics Society, 37, 725-729.

10. Breitbart W, Rosenfeld B, Roth A, Smith MJ, Cohen K & Passik, S (1997). The memorial delirium assessment scale. Journal of Pain and Symptom Management, 13, 128-137.

11. Ewing JA (1984). Detecting alcoholism. The CAGE questionnaire. The Journal of the American Medical Association, 252, 1905-1907.

12. Puchalski CM & Romer AL (2000). Taking a spiritual history allows clinicians to understand patients more fully. Journal of Palliative Medicine, 3, 129-137. FICA Questions Reproduced with permission from the author. © Christina M. Puchalski, MD, FACP, Director, The George Washington Institute of Spirituality and Health Associate Prof of Medicine, Healthcare Sciences, The George Washington University School of Medine; Associate Professor of Health Management and Leadership, The George Washington University School of Public Health School of Medicine and Health Sciences; 2131 K St NW Suite 510; Washington, DC 20037; www.gwish.org.

* The NCCN Guidelines are a work in progress that will be refined as often as new significant data becomes available.

The NCCN Guidelines are a statement of consensus of its authors regarding their views of currently accepted approaches to treatment. Any clinician seeking to apply or consult any NCCN guideline is expected to use independent medical judgement in the context of individual clinical circumstances to determine any patinet's care or treatment. The National Comprehensive Cancer Network makes no warranties of any kind whatsoever regarding their content, use or application and disclaims any responsibility for their application or use in any way.

3 Psychiatric Emergencies

How does an oncology team handle a psychiatric emergency when a psychiatric consultant is not available? First priority: safety of the patient and anyone else in danger.

Table 3.1 Who are the Patients who Require Urgent Management?

- Patients who are *violent or suicidal*
- Patients who have *questionable competency* to refuse appropriate urgent treatment
- Patients who are *restless, pacing, threatening, demanding, and/or pulling out tubes*

Table 3.2 Management Principles for Psychiatric Emergencies

How can the patient be safe, watched, and assessed? The answer depends on the setting.	• In the *hospital*, call a security officer. Does the patient need an order for one-to-one constant observation for safety? • In the *clinic*, is there sufficient staff or assistance to monitor and control the patient's behavior? Call 911? • If at *home*, can family bring the patient to clinic or Emergency Room? If not, call 911 or police to take the patient to the nearest emergency room.
Obtain information from chart, staff, and family as quickly as possible.	• What is the behavior creating the emergency? • Assess the mental status of the patient: disoriented, delusional, hallucinating, or psychotic? • What is the timeframe for the change in behavior? • What is the medical status of the patient? • Is there any history of alcohol or substance use or abuse? • Has the patient been agitated, confused, suicidal or violent before? • What is the working differential diagnosis?
Take charge.	• The key to handling a psychiatric emergency is to *identify one person who is in charge*, preferably the oncologist. Emotions are high, and a single individual should direct the management of the emergency. Your calm stance is critical to safety for the patient, family, staff and other bystanders who are frightened by disruptive behavior. • Enlist some one the patient trusts, a staff member or family member, to reassure the patient. • Give clear and concise instructions to all involved.

(Continued, next page)

Table 3.2   Management Principles (continued)

Work-up	• Assume a medical cause of agitation or confusion until proven otherwise. • Agitation or confusion may signal a medical emergency.

Being prepared	• Develop a "psychiatric code" procedure for psychiatric emergencies and practice it periodically with the team.
	• Useful phone numbers should be on hand and easily available:
	  • Hospital Security, 911, or police • Chaplaincy
	  • Psychiatrist on call • Social Work
	  • Emergency Room • Psychiatric hospital admission

Physical restraint	• Enough well-trained staff are necessary to secure each limb. Four security guards or strong staff members may be needed to escort the patient. • Patients with cancer must be physically restrained with care because of their frailty, clotting impairments, and fragile bones. • *Physical restraints* are used as briefly as possible, usually with either 2-point (arms) or 4-point (arms and legs) restraint devices. • *Four-point restraints* require checks every 15 minutes; a physician's order must be renewed every 4 hours. The patient remains under one-to-one constant observation status while 4-point restraints are in use. • Inject *a tranquilizer*, e.g. *haloperidol* (Haldol®) as the patient is put into restraints if the cause of agitation is clear and not from an undiagnosed medical problem. • Psychotropic medications should not be used as chemical restraints. • Vital signs should be checked frequently and restraint sites rotated. • Each institution may have distinct legal policies.

Medication to tranquilize (cf. Chapter 4, Tables 4.4 and 4.6)	***Antipsychotics (preferred)*** - *haloperidol* (Haldol®), *chlorpromazine* (Thorazine®), *perphenazine* (Trilafon®)
	Atypical antipsychotics - *ziprasidone* (Geodon®), *risperidone* (Risperdal®), *quetiapine* (Seroquel®), *olanzapine* (Zyprexa®), *ziprasidone* (Geodon®)
	Benzodiazepines - *alprazolam* (Xanax®), *diazepam* (Valium®), *lorazepam* (Ativan®)
	  • Benzodiazepines in excess can cause intoxication and delirium but are useful for acute sedation; for delirium, benzodiazepines should only be used with antipsychotics.
	  • After the patient is calm, the medical evaluation needs to be expedited.
	  • Continue to observe the patient closely for safety and for the need of more medication.
	  • Tranquilizers are sometimes continued up to seven days if the cause has not been reversed.
	  • May be slowly tapered.

Table 3.3   Differential Diagnosis for Agitation or Confusion

- Pulmonary embolus
- Sepsis
- Uncontrolled pain
- Delirium
- Metabolic abnormalities (hypoglycemia, hypercalcemia, hypoxia)
- Intoxication with narcotics or benzodiazepines
- Side effects of medications like restlessness (akathisia) from anti-nausea medications
- Mania or psychosis from steroids
- Brain metastases
- Alcohol or benzodiazepine withdrawal
- Drug intoxication
- Acute grief reactions
- Hysterical dramatic threats from a patient with personality disorder

Interventions

Several steps may be taken to calm the patient. If needed, medication may be used to tranquilize the patient. An algorithm for medication is provided in Figure 3.1, and guidance on application of the algorithim may be found in Table 3.5

Table 3.4   Calming the Agitated Patient

- Start by talking to the patient to calm excited behavior.
- Isolate the patient away from other patients and visitors in the hospital or clinic.
- If in the hospital, escort the patient to a quiet room, with security, if needed, away from other patients.
- Determine whether family or friends are helping to calm the patient or agitating further. Enlist their help if they understand the situation.
- Identify the staff member the patient trusts (e.g., male, female, older, younger, and trusted before); ask staff members who are the target of the patient's paranoia not to participate temporarily.
- Offer the 'non-choice choice': Tell the patient they may choose what to do. "You can take the haloperidol (Haldol®) liquid, a calming medication, by mouth or we can give you an injection of Haldol®, either in a muscle or by the IV. Which would you rather have?"
- Or you may say, "We can all walk to your room and you can lie down, or the security guards can escort you to your room." Each time, you offer a more or less intrusive and coercive choice. The more rational the patient's thinking, the more likely he/she will choose the less intrusive option.
- Calm, concise explanations help the patient to cooperate. Allow the patient to express his concerns and frustrations in order to reduce the fears and lack of cooperation.

Figure 3.1 Algorithm for Medicating Agitation*

MEDICATION:	Haloperidol	OR SWITCH TO →	Chlorpromazine	OR USE/ SWITCH TO ←→	Olanzapine
APPROXIMATE DAILY DOSE:	0.5 - 10 mg Q 2 - 12 hr		25 - 50 mg IV Q 4 h - 12 hr if increased sedation desired OR if haloperidol or olanzapine regimen is not tolerated		2.5 - 5 mg if EPS is a concern or if increased sedation desired OR if haloperidol or chlorpromazine regimen is not tolerated
ROUTE:	IV, IM, PO		IV, IM, PO		PO, IM or Zydis wafer
NEED TO WATCH FOR:	Extrapyramidal symptoms (EPS), EKG If EPS is present, add benztropine 0.5 - 1 mg If increased sedation desired, add lorazepam 0.5 - 2 mg		EKG abnormalities, BP, Liver function tests, Anticholinergic side effects, Hypotension		Anticholinergic side effects If EPS is present, add benztropine 0.5 - 1 mg or diphenhydramine 25 - 50 mg

Discussion of each medication is provided in Table 3.5 below.

Table 3.5 Psychopharmacological Management*

haloperidol (Haldol®) - neuroleptic agent potent dopamine blocker; **drug of choice**; effective in diminishing agitation, paranoia and fear

Check vital signs and obtain an EKG. Start with low doses (0.5 mg -2 mg dose IV, and double the dose every 30 to 60 minutes until agitation is decreased). Parenteral doses are approximately twice as potent as oral doses.

lorazepam (Ativan®) - should not be given alone when delirium causes agitation, since it may increase confusion

Common strategy is to add parenteral *lorazepam* (0.5 -2 mg IV) to a regimen of *haloperidol*, which may help to rapidly sedate the agitated delirious patient.

chlorpromazine (Thorazine®) - for a very agitated or combative patient who does not respond

Intravenously (cf. Figure 3.1 above), but be alert to potential hypotensive and anticholinergic side effects.

Newer *atypical neuroleptic drugs* have fewer risks of dystonia, Parkinsonism, and restlessness, but may cause postural hypotension and sedation.
- *olanzapine* (Zyprexa®, Zydis®)
- *risperidone* (Risperdal®)
- *quetiapine* (Seroquel®)
- *ziprasidone* (Geodon®)

Elderly or frail patients require lower doses of these medications. Added risks of sedation and postural hypotension in older patients with dementia. May be given intramuscularly. *Olanzapine* is available in orally disintegrating tablets (Zydis®) and intramuscularly. *Risperidone* (Risperdal®) is available in orally disintegrating tablets and liquid. These medications can be immediately calming.

* Cf. Chapter 4, Table 4.6.

Management of a Suicidal Emergency

Assessment of Risk

Suicidal thoughts are frightening for the patient, family and the medical staff. Figuring out if someone is in acute danger of self-destructive behavior is not always easy. The patient may be thinking, "If it gets bad enough, then I will kill myself." Most patients do not want to die and probably will not harm themselves, but wish to share their frustration and fears about their situation. (Cf. Chapter 6, Mood Disorders.)

Examples of expressions of suicide which are not usually accompanied by high risk
- "I've dealt with this illness for so many years, I don't think I can go through another procedure and would rather die."
- "This may be a new diagnosis, but it is Cancer. If the pain ever gets bad enough, I will kill myself."

Examples of expressions with greater suicidal risk
- "This pain is unbearable. There's no way I can go on living like this." The patient has a gun at home.
- "Everyone would be better off without me." The patient is stockpiling pills.

The seriousness of the patient's intentions should be explored. Suicide occurs in patients with depression, severe anxiety, panic, intoxication, or delirium. **It is important to ask if the patient has made a definite plan.**

Table 3.6 Questions to Ask Patients or Family When Assessing Suicidal Risk

Acknowledge that these are common thoughts that can be discussed.	• Most patients with cancer have passing thoughts about suicide, such as "I might do something if it gets bad enough." Have you ever had thoughts like that? • Have you had any thoughts of not wanting to live? • Have you had those thoughts in the past few days?
Assess Level of Risk.	• Do you have thoughts about wanting to end your life? How? • Do you have a plan? • Do you have any strong social supports? • Do you have pills stockpiled at home? • Do you own or have access to a weapon?
Obtain Prior History.	• Have you ever had a psychiatric disorder, suffered from depression, or made a suicide attempt? • Is there a family history of suicide?

(continued, next page)

Table 3.6   Questions to Ask When Assessing Suicidal Risk (continued)

Identify Substance Abuse.	• Have you had a problem with alcohol or drugs?
Identify Bereavement.	• Have you lost anyone close to you recently?
Identify Medical Predictors of Risk.	• Do you have pain that is not being relieved? • How has the disease affected your life? • How is your memory and concentration? • Do you feel hopeless? • What do you plan for the future?

Table 3.7   Interventions for Suicidal Patient

For patient whose suicidal threat is seen as serious	• Provide constant observation and further assessment. • Dangerous objects like guns or intoxicants should be removed from the room or home. • The risk for suicidal behavior should be communicated to family members.
For patient who is not deemed acutely suicidal and is medically stabilized	• The patient should agree to call when feeling overwhelmed, making a contract with the physician to talk about suicidal thoughts in the future rather than to act on them.
For inpatients	• Room searches should be carried out to make sure there are no means available for self-destructive behavior. • The patient should be under constant observation from the time suicidal thoughts are expressed.
For severely suicidal outpatients whose suicidal thoughts are not acutely caused by their medical condition or medication	• Psychiatric hospitalization is warranted, either by voluntary or involuntary means. • A psychiatrist can assist in making these arrangements. Document medical action and reasoning in the crisis.

Management of Refusal of Treatment or Demand to Leave

Another frequent emergency is the patient who wants to leave the hospital against medical advice, or who refuses medical or surgical procedures (ie, lumbar punctures, placement of central catheters). The oncologist may have to evaluate the patient's capacity to make decisions about medical care.

Table 3.8   Interventions to Evaluate Treatment Refusal

- Sit down with the patient to find out what he understands about his predicament.
- Do a mental status examination and determine if there is compromise of cognition.
- Until the patient's cognition and judgment are assessed, he can be detained.
- Assess judgment and insight in relation to the specific decision about the procedure or situation.
- Ask, "Does the patient have the capacity (understanding) to make a decision about refusing this MRI scan, or lumbar puncture?"
- The patient may be able to understand the issues related to some decisions and not to others.
- The gravity of the decision to refuse treatment, the life-threatening nature or potential benefit of a decision, guides the depth of the evaluation of a patient's understanding of the illness, treatment recommendations, and consequences of refusing. In complex situations, a psychiatric consultation or an ethics committee review may be helpful.

References

1. Allen MA (Ed.). (2002). *Emergency Psychiatry.* Washington, DC: American Psychiatric Publishing Inc.

2. Bostwick JM & Levenson JL (2005). Suicidality. In JL Levenson (Ed.), *The American Psychiatric Publishing Textbook of Psychosomatic Medicine* (pp. 219-234). Washington, DC: American Psychiatric Publishing Inc.

3. Moore DP & Jefferson JW (2004). *Handbook of Medical Psychiatry.* St. Louis, MO: Mosby.

4. Stern TA, Fricchione GL, Cassem NH, Jellinek MS & Rosenbaum JF (Eds.). (2004). *Massachusetts General Hospital Handbook of General Hospital Psychiatry* (5th ed.). PA: Mosby.

5. Onike CU & Lyketsos CG (2005). Aggression and violence. In JL Levenson (Ed.), *The American Psychiatric Publishing Textbook of Psychosomatic Medicine* (pp. 171-191). Washington, DC: American Psychiatric Publishing Inc.

6. Roth AJ & Breitbart W (1996). Psychiatric emergencies in terminally ill cancer patients. *Hematology/Oncology Clinics of North America, 10,* 235-259.

4   Pharmacological Interventions

Psychotropic drugs are highly effective for treatment of anxiety, depression, agitation, and confusion in cancer patients. Oncologists often use psychotropic medications to alleviate these symptoms. These principles will guide more effective use of these psychotropic drugs. The major categories of drugs: anti-depressants, anti-anxiety medications and major tranquilizers (antipsychotics, neuroleptics) are outlined below. Specific psychiatric diagnoses and their psychopharmacological management are outlined in Chapter 6 and in the sections of Chapter 9 devoted to unique problems associated with each type of cancer.

Table 4.1   Psychotropic Drugs by Class

Antidepressants: Selective Serotonin Reuptake Inhibitors (SSRI) and Newer Antidepressants (Cf. Table 4.2.)	• Benefits for major depressive disorder and chronic, recurrent anxiety depend on daily adherence and clinical assessments at 28 days or longer. Sleep, restlessness, and hopelessness improve gradually over several weeks to 2 months.
	• Also used for anxiety disorders, recurrent panic attacks, obsessive-compulsive disorders.
	• Because of the co-morbidities of cancer patients, doses can be started low to minimize side effects and to allow the patient to become comfortable with this additional drug. "Start low; go slow" is the dictum, particularly for fearful patients. When first started, they may be energizing or increase anxiety. This activation can be distressing in itself and can be minimized by reducing the dose. It is helpful to assess side effects often during the first two weeks.
	• Depression carries with it a risk of suicide. It is essential to monitor for suicidal thoughts. Sometimes patients develop energy before hopelessness increases, and this mix contributes to risk of suicide.
	• Nausea, indigestion, and softer stools from serotonin agonists are generally mild when compared to the gastrointestinal side effects of chemotherapy or abdominal radiation therapy. Patients on medicines that cause constipation, such as opioids, may welcome bowel stimulation. The antidote for the mild nausea of serotonin-agonist drugs like SSRIs is a 5-HT3 antagonist like ondansetron.
	• A mild withdrawal syndrome can occur when short half-life drugs, like *paroxetine* (Paxil®) or *venlafaxine* (Effexor®) are stopped abruptly. Most antidepressants should be tapered slowly over several weeks. Withdrawal symptoms are not serious, but include malaise, dizziness, and lightening-like pains.

(continued, next page)

Table 4.1 Psychotropic Drugs by Class (continued)

SSRIs and Newer Antidepressants (continued) (Cf. Table 4.2.)	• *Venlafaxine* (Effexor®) and *duloxetine* (Cymbalta®) are both usful for treatment of neuropathic pain. • *Paroxetine* (Paxil®) and *venlafaxine* (Effexor®) have been helpful for hot flashes.
Antidepressants: Tricyclics (Cf. Table 4.3.)	• Besides antidepressant effects, these medications also have benefits for neuropathic pain at lower doses than the doses used for depression. • May cause postural hypotension because they block alpha adrenergic receptors. • They are also antihistaminic and cause sedation. • They prolong conduction from the His bundle to the ventricle so are used with caution in patients with bundle branch block. • They share side effects of dry mouth, urinary hesitancy, and constipation with opioids. • Monitor for dry mouth, blurry vision, constipation, urinary retention, all anticholinergic side effects.
Anti-anxiety/ Sedative Drugs (Cf. Table 4.4.)	• *Benzodiazapines* are often used for nausea (particularly *lorazepam* (Ativan®). Patients may have a supply at home for use with chemotherapy. Lorazapam is a good choice with medium half-life for anxiety. • Good choices for anticipatory anxiety, claustrophobia, panic attacks. When panic attacks are recurrent, serotonin reuptake inhibitors are a better choice. • Avoid stopping abruptly (even if used as needed only); discontinuation can cause rebound anxiety and jitteriness. • Patients become tolerant; the same dose may not be as potent after a while, so drug holidays may be an option to decrease tolerance. • Patients who drink alcohol regularly may abuse benzodiazapines.
Hypnotics (Cf. Table 4.5.)	• Hypnotics help patients to fall asleep but last briefly. Antidepressant medications may be better for broken sleep, early morning wakening, and hot flashes. • Consider sleep apnea as a reason for poor sleep in those who snore. • When hypnotics are stopped abruptly, patients will have temporary trouble sleeping. • Patients who have confusional states and insomnia are better managed with anti-psychotics.

(continued, next page)

Table 4.1   Psychotropic Drugs by Class (continued)

Anti-psychotic medications: Major tranquilizers (Cf. Table 4.6.)	• *haloperidol* (Haldol®) is the gold standard for treatment of delirium or encephalopathy. It has been used for many years and is available in flexible dosing formulations (oral tablets, liquid, intravenous, intramuscularly).
	• Repeated doses can cause extrapyramidal side effects like restlessness, Parkinsonism (tremor, bradykinesia, tardive dyskinesia) that can easily be mistaken for anxiety or depression.
	• Antiemetics like *prochlorperazine* (Compazine®) or *metoclopramide* (Reglan®) block dopamine and give similar side effects. When these drugs are added to dopamine blocking anti-psychotics, the risk of similar side effects is greater.
	• The newer atypical tranquilizers like *olanzapine* (Zyprexa®) and *risperidone* (Risperdal®) have a lower risk of extrapyramidal side effects, but they may cause restlessness and Parkinsonism. Use with caution in older patients with dementia.
	• When using tranquilizers that can cause postural hypotension are used, especially *risperidone* (Risperdal®), pay attention to other conditions or medications that reduce blood pressure, such as anti-hypertensives.
	• *Olanzapine* (Zyprexa®) and *quetiapine* (Seroquel®) are antihistaminic and somewhat anticholinergic, so they can cause sedation. *Olanzapine* causes weight gain.
	• These drugs improve cognition in the delirious, confused patient and do not simply sedate.
	• If the patient is lethargic due to delirium, antipsychotic medications may improve alert concentration.
	• Severe agitation may require both major tranquilizers and benzodiazepines.

Table 4.2 Antidepressants: Selective Serotonin Reuptake Inhibitors (SSRI) and Newer Antidepressants

Generic	Brand Names	Starting Dose	Maximal Dose (24h)	Sedating ✓	Forms Available	Take Note*
bupropion	Wellbutrin®, Zyban®	75 mg	300 mg		SR (bid) XL	Use <150 mg per dose except XL; fewer sexual side effects; risk of seizures; also for smoking cessation
citalopram	Celexa®	10 mg	40 mg		soltabs†	†New form in 2006
duloxetine	Cymbalta®	20 mg	60 mg	✓		Also for neuropathic pain; taper slowly
escitalopram	Lexapro®	5 mg	20 mg			Isomer of citalopram
fluoxetine	Prozac®, Sarafem®	5 mg	60 mg			Moderate benefit for hot flashes, premenstrual syndrome
mirtazapine	Remeron®	15 mg	45 mg	✓✓	soltabs	Very sedating; stimulates appetite
paroxetine	Paxil®	5 mg	40 mg	✓		Also for hot flashes; slow taper
sertraline	Zoloft®	25 mg	200 mg			
trazodone	Desyrel®	50 mg	300 mg	✓		Primarily for insomnia
venlafaxine	Effexor®	25-37.5mg	375 mg		XR QD	Also for hot flashes and neuropathic pain; slow taper

Table 4.3 Antidepressants: Tricyclics

Generic	Brand Name	Starting Dose	Maximal Dose (24h)	Take Note*
amitriptyline	Elavil®	10 mg	300 mg	25-50 mg for pain
desipramine	Norpramin®	10 mg	300 mg	
doxepin	Sinequan®	10 mg	150 mg	Very antihistaminic; sedating; also for itching
imipramine	Tofranil®	10 mg	300 mg	
nortriptyline	Pamelor®	10 mg	150 mg	25 mg for pain

* Cf. Table 4.1 on pages 26 - 27.

Table 4.4   Anti-anxiety/Sedative Drugs

Generic	Brand Name	Starting Dose	Maximal Dose (24 h)	Half-Life Short	Med	Long	Take Note*
alprazolam	Xanax®	0.25 mg	4 mg	X (XR available)			Short-acting; difficult to stop
clonazepam	Klonopin®	0.25 mg	4 mg			X	Can use *bid* or *tid* for continuous coverage; wafer available (0.125-2 mg)
diazepam	Valium®	2 mg	20 mg		X		Rapidly absorbed, but long half-life
lorazepam	Ativan®	0.25 mg	5 mg	X			Widely used anti-emetic; sleep aid
midazolam	Versed®	†	†	X			† At anesthesiologist's discretion

Table 4.5   Hypnotics

Generic	Brand Name	Starting Dose	Maximal Dose (24 h)	Half-Life Short	Med	Take Note*
eszopiclone	Lunesta®	1 mg	3 mg	X		For sleep
oxazapam	Serax®	10 mg	30 mg	X		For sleep, also for alcohol withdrawal
temazepam	Restoril®	7.5 mg	30 mg		X	For insomnia
triazolam	Halcion®	0.125 mg	0.5 mg	X		For insomnia
zaleplon	Sonata®	5 mg	20 mg	X		For sleep
zolpidem	Ambien®	2.5 mg	10 mg	X		For sleep, technically non-benzodiazapine but shares properties (dependence, withdrawal)

Cf. Table 4.1 on page 27.

Table 4.6   Anti-psychotic medications: Major tranquilizers

Generic	Brand Name	Starting Dose	Maximal Dose	Forms Available	Administration Routes	Take Note*
chlorpormazine	Thorazine®	10 mg	200 mg			Parenteral; postural hypotension; sedation; hiccups
haloperidol	Haldol®	0.25 mg	30 mg	I.V., P.O.,	I.V., P.O.	Anti-emetic; risk of extrapyramidal side effects; parenteral; liquid
olanzapine	Zyprexa® (Zydis®)	2.5 mg	20 mg	Wafer, P.O.		Wafer form (Zydis®); weight gain; antiemetic sedation; long term risk of diabetes; can cause restlessness
perphenazine	Trilafon®	2 mg	32mg			
quetiapine	Seroquel®	25 mg	500 mg		P.O.	Antihistamine associated somnolence; 5-hour half-life
risperidone	Risperdal®	0.25 mg	8 mg			Postural hypotension; smaller risk of Parkinson's than typical agents

References

1. Stern TA, Fricchione GL, Cassem NH, Jellinek MS, Rosenbaum JF (Eds.). (2004). *Massachusetts general hospital handbook of general hospital psychiatry* (5th ed.). PA: Mosby.

2. Holland JC (Ed.). (1998). *Psycho-Oncology*. New York: Oxford University Press.

* Cf. Table 4.1 on page 28.

5 Psychological Non-pharmacological Interventions

Understanding the Patient Experience

The primary oncology team is the keystone for assisting the patient and family in coping (cf. Figure 1.1 on page 2).[1,2] Good communication, mutual respect and trust between oncologist and patient are critical. These are combined with clear information about the illness, help to mobilize family resources, and control of such symptoms as insomnia and poor appetite. This chapter outlines some easy and helpful brief interventions and suggests referrals to support groups and advocacy organizations in the patient's community for added support. Support groups or advocacy organizations are particularly helpful for patients who have few personal or social resources.

Evidenced-Based Interventions[3]

This chapter outlines six evidenced-based interventions that the primary oncology team can use readily for managing mild to moderate forms of distress encountered in daily practice, or they may refer patients to community resources to receive these interventions:

- Cognitive Behavioral Therapy (CBT)
- Stress reduction exercises
- Problem-solving techniques: COPE
- Exercise
- Support groups
- Complementary therapies

Cognitive Behavioral Therapy Techniques[4,5]

Cognitive-behavioral interventions are mental and behavioral techniques designed to modify specific emotional, behavioral and social problems, and alleviate anxiety, depression, and distress. Fears that arise with a cancer diagnosis create a chronic state of uncertainty. Therefore, the goal of CBT is to enhance the sense of personal control and self-efficacy despite the illness.

Cognitive techniques are applied to thoughts, images, and attitudes. For example, guided mental imagery is a cognitive process.

Cognitive Coping

Cognitive techniques for coping with anxiety, depression, pain and distress increase relaxation and reduce the intensity and distressing qualities of the stressful experience. Similar techniques have been successful for coping with pain, nausea and vomiting.

The following are samples of cognitive coping techniques:

Distraction:
- *Inattention*—imagine yourself sunbathing on the beach
- *Mental Distraction*—do mental arithmetic, memorize a poem
- *Behavioral Task Distraction*—read, write, hobby-related activity; music therapy; hypnosis

Focusing: To reduce anxiety and distress (pain, fatigue, nausea) patients are asked to: Imagine a painful sensation such as heat radiating from an oven.
- Visualize the temperature dial and gradually turn down the heat and then turn off the oven.
- Visualize themselves as an injured football player continuing to play despite discomfort. [This is best related to patients' own experiences—it could be ballet, swimming, etc]
- Imagine a painful body part as not being a part of their body, thereby "disassociating" the painful part.

All of these methods change the focus of attention. They modify the natural tendency for "hypervigilance," overconcern about a minor symptom. They change meanings, beliefs, and habits of thinking. Often pain is worse until patients are told that the pain does not represent spread of cancer. Patients are also told that relief will not be immediate; therefore, the patient will not pay too close attention immediately after treatment and diminish the positive effects.

Cognitive Reframing

Patients are asked to think about problems so that they become more tolerable. If they feel overwhelmed by the thought of two months of chemotherapy, ask them to reframe the treatment plan into one week at a time, creating time blocks that are more tolerable.

If they feel guilty about requiring too much of the family's time and attention, they may recognize the positive benefit of the opportunity for closeness.

Patients who view crying as a weakness, may be able to see its benefit for feeling refreshed and relieved.

Cognitive Modification

Note how the patients' ways of thinking make their distress greater. These cognitive processes represent beliefs and reactions that are based on personal experiences. The caregivers' recognition that the patient suffers from his pattern of thinking may count. For example, when the patient says, "*I know my doctor is giving up on me. He didn't tell me how I was doing and I know that means things are bad*," the staff may empathize with how negative he feels when he is not reassured by the doctor. The understanding of distress can be transmitted without the patient being falsely or constantly reassured.

Table 5.1   Stress Reduction and Relaxation Exercises

These are designed to achieve mental and physical relaxation. Any method that reduces tension is useful.

Passive Relaxation	Focusing attention on sensations of warmth and relaxation in various parts of the body with verbal suggestions and pleasant imagery.
Progressive Muscle Relaxation	Actively tense and relax muscle groups, and focus on the sensations. Find a comfortable position and sequentially tighten and relax muscle groups. Start with hands, arms, feet and legs, torso, head and the whole body.
Meditation	Chant or repeat a word or rehearse a specific sentence to focus attention away from distressing feelings and thoughts. Breathe gently in and out as the word, phrase or sentence is repeated. For example, breathe in slowly (counting 1, 2) and on the out breath slowly say, "Relax" (counting 1, 2).
Mindfulness Meditation	Focus the mind on something specific (like breath) with intention. Attend to the present moment and let go of the past and the future. Fifteen to twenty minutes of this exercise are quite refreshing and relaxing. The steps are: • Chose a quiet place; • Sit or lay comfortably; • Close your eyes; • Take a deep breath and let it out slowly (repeat 2 or 3 times); • Focus attention on the breath—gently going in and out; • As thoughts enter, just watch them and let them go like clouds or birds moving across the sky; • Return your focus to breathing in and out; • Sit quietly for a few moments; • When you are ready to stop, take a deep breath, gently stretch and open your eyes.
Biofeedback	Relaxation of specific tense muscles or chronically aroused autonomic functions.
Guided Imagery	Find an image that is associated with a feeling of well-being and peace. Examples: A mountain stream with rushing waters or biking on a beach at sunset.

Problem-Solving Approach

The COPE Model makes tracking problem-solving much easier.[6,7] Houts proposed a new conceptual model that focuses on cancer. The acronym COPE summarizes the four essential elements of the problem-solving motivational approach shown in the table.

Table 5.2 COPE Model

Creativity	Creativity is necessary to overcome obstacles in patient and family members, and to manage the emotional and interpersonal problems that result from a chronic illness. It is also necessary to enable the family to see problems and solutions in new way.
Optimism	Optimisim is necessary to face the family attitudes and expectations regarding the problem-solving process. Family needs realistic optimism. While they recognize the seriousness of problems, they need to see that new solutions are possible.
Planning	Families develop plans to implement medical instructions, and plans to address the emotional challenges associated with cancer therapies.
Expert Information	Guidance from health care professionals on how to manage physical and emotional problems due to cancer and its related treatments encourages a sense of control and confidence.

Physical Exercise[8,9]

Health benefits of physical exercise are:

Increased energy	Decreased fatigue
Improved sleep	Decreased pain
Improved blood & lymph flow	Decreased depression
Improved immune function	Decreased anxiety

Exercise is of benefit for both physical and emotional health, despite any level of fatigue. The quick reference chart provides a way to assess current activity/energy level, and recommended mild exercise for the amount of time that corresponds to their energy level.

A quick reference chart for physical exercise recommendations is provided in Table 5.3.

Table 5.3   Physical Exercise Recommendation - Quick Reference Chart*

Screening Item for Activity/ Energy Level	Activity Level (Energy equiv. 1-10)	Recommended Exercise Time Goal	Recommended Exercise Type
	15 minutes (1-2 out of 10)	2 minutes - 2 times per day (or 4 minutes total or less)	Mild, Slow, Gentle, Low Impact
	30 minutes (3-4 out of 10)	4 minutes - 2 times per day (or 8 minutes total or less)	Walking, yoga
Today I have enough energy to do my activities of daily living (work, chores, leisure) for:	2 hours (5-6 out of 10)	6 minutes - 2 times per day (or 12 minutes total or less)	Talk Test —Exercise at pace you can go and still speak in full sentences without getting out of breath
	4 hours (7-8 out of 10)	9 minutes - 2 times per day (or 18 minutes total or less)	
	8 hours (9-10 out of 10)	13 minutes - 2 times per day (or 26 minutes total or less)	

* Avoid movement that causes pain, difficulty breathing, or any problems with existing medical conditions. Exercise enough to feel more energized, and avoid exercise that leaves you feeling more fatigued.

Support Groups

Over the last 25 years, extensive research has been done on the positive effects of support groups as a method of coping with cancer, and improving quality of life.[10-14] This research has shown that support groups help to improve mood and the perception of pain, especially in those initially more distressed.

Community-based cancer support programs like The Wellness Community (www.thewellnesscommunity.org), Gilda's Club (www.gildasclub.org), CancerCare (www.cancercare.org), and disease specific organizations like Lung Cancer Alliance (www.lca.org) play critical supportive roles which are part of advocacy organizations and offer free services to patients and families. In nonrandomized studies of community-based cancer support programs, participants generally rate their experiences as positive and beneficial. In a study done at The Wellness Community (TWC) with Stanford University, support groups in the community that encourage preparing for the worst while hoping for the best have been shown to reduce cancer patients' overall distress. There is a growing body of research indicating that Internet support groups like those provided by TWC, CancerCare, and the American Cancer Society (ACS) may also be effective to decrease depression and negative reaction to pain while increasing zest for life and spirituality. These groups are especially useful for those who may prefer the anonymity of the Internet, live too far away or are too ill to attend a face-to-face group.

Keep a list of available support groups in the community to provide easy referral to the appropriate group. Some are organized by site or stage of cancer. In general, the more homogeneous the group members are the more they share the same problems. Groups facilitators are usually trained counselors. Some patients do not find groups helpful or are afraid to try them. Referral for individual counselors in the community should be kept handy for easy reference.

If counselors are not known in the patients' community, call the American Psychosocial Oncology Society (APOS) Helpline 1-866-APOS-4-HELP (1-866-276-7443) which provides referrals to local counselors trained in oncology and counseling, or local support groups. (Cf. Chapter 10.)

Complementary Treatments

These are treatments adjunctive to conventional medical treatment that help to control symptoms and enhance quality of life.[2] Examples are:

- **Music/Dance Therapy:** A professional therapist engages patients individually or in groups in active or passive musical/dance experiences. Music/dance can have a mood altering effect, as well as an indirect relaxing effect through the diversion of attention from stress- provoking stimuli.
- **Art Therapy:** A therapist uses art forms to help patients express anger, loss, fears, vulnerability, and depression. Art therapy's premise is that emotions that would or could not be expressed in words can be expressed in images thereby reducing stress and isolation.
- **Journaling:** Expressive writing in the form of a journal or notebook especially about upsetting experiences can have a positive effect on negative or traumatic experiences.

References

1. Henke Yarbro C, Goodman M & Hansen Frogge M (Eds.). (2004). *Cancer symptom management* (3rd ed., pp. 24, 52, 89, 133, 466-467, 470). Sudbury, MA: Jones and Bartlett Publishers.

2. Holland J & Lewis S (2000). *The human side of cancer: Living with hope, coping with uncertainty.* New York: HarperCollins.

3. Fawzy FI, Fawzy NW, Hyun CS, Elashoff R, Guthrie D, Fahey JL, et al. (1993). Malignant melanoma. Effects of an early structured psychiatric intervention, coping, and affective state on recurrence and survival 6 years later. *Archives of General Psychiatry, 50,* 681-689.

4. Fishman, B & Loscalzo, M (1987). Cognitive-behavioral interventions in management of cancer pain: Principles and application. *Medical Clinics of North America*, 71, 271-287.

5. Loscalzo M & Jacobsen P (1990). Practical behavioral approaches to the effective management of pain and distress. *Journal of Psychosocial Oncology*, 8, 139-169.

6. Houts PS, Nezu AM, Nezu CM & Bucher JA (1996). The prepared family caregiver: A problem-solving approach to family caregiver education. *Patient Education & Counseling*, 27, 63-73.

7. Nezu AM, Nezu, CM, Houts P, Friedman S & Faddis S (1999). Relevance of problem-solving therapy to psychosocial oncology. *Journal of Psychosocial Oncology*, 16(3/4), 5-26.

8. Galvao DA & Newton RU (2005). Review of exercise intervention studies in cancer patients. *Journal of Clinical Oncology*, 23, 899-909.

9. Sharkey BJ (1990). *Physiology of Fitness* (3rd ed.). Champaign, IL: Human Kinetics.

10. Cordova MJ, Giese-Davis J, Golant M, Kronnenwetter C, Chang V, McFarlin S, et al. (2003). Mood disturbance in community cancer support groups. The role of emotional suppression and fighting spirit. *Journal of Psychosomatic Research*, 55, 461-467.

11. Glajchen M & Magen R (1995). Evaluating process, outcome, and satisfaction in community-based cancer support research. *Social Work with Groups*, 18(1), 27-40.

12. Goodwin P, Leszcz M, Ennis M, Koopmans J, Vincent L, Guther H, et al. (2001). The effect of group psychosocial support on survival in metastatic breast cancer. *New England Journal of Medicine*, 345, 1719-1726.

13. Lieberman M, Golant M, Giese-Davis J, Winzlenberg A, Benjamin H, Humphreys K, et al. (2003). Electronic support groups for breast carcinoma: A clinical trial of effectiveness. *Cancer*, 97, 920-925.

14. Spiegel D, Bloom JR & Yalom I (1981). Group support for patients with metastatic cancer. A randomized outcome study. *Archives of General Psychiatry*, 38, 527-533.

6 Common Psychiatric Disorders

Anxiety Disorders
Introduction
Cancer patients are vulnerable to anxiety in all phases of the disease experience, from screening for risk in those without documented disease, through active treatment, to life as a cancer survivor or to end-stage disease in those who do not survive. Low intensity anxiety is often self-limited and may be contained fairly easily. Anxiety is not always maladaptive and sometimes has beneficial effects (e.g., increased motivation to stop smoking, compliance with treatment recommendations, etc). More persistent or intense anxiety can significantly affect a patient's ability to function in all aspects of life and interfere with treatment. Chronic anxiety may result from serious medical pathology. In the general population anxiety is defined as pathological if it is disproportionate to the level of threat to the individual. It is difficult to make such an assignment in the face of a cancer diagnosis, which is almost always threatening. Other criteria (symptoms that are unacceptable regardless of threat, and which disrupt normal function) should be given the most emphasis.[1] Prevalence estimates of pathological anxiety in cancer vary greatly, with rates using well-defined criteria approaching 30% in some studies.[2,3]

Table 6.1 Signs and Symptoms of Anxiety

Psychological	• Worry, apprehension, fear, and sadness • Patient may be able to identify focus or source of these symptoms • Often non-specific and "free floating" • Crying spells, ruminations • Typical complaint (especially at night): inability to "turn off" one's thoughts
Physical	• Tachycardia and tachypnea • Tremor, diaphoresis, nausea, dry mouth, insomnia, and anorexia
May be intermittent; increasing over hours or days	• In response to a stressor (e.g., anticipation of pending diagnostic tests or procedures) with resolution if/when the stressor passes

(continued, next page)

Table 6.1   Signs and Symptoms of Anxiety (continued)

May be persistent and pervasive through the day	• Typical of primary anxiety disorders • Co-morbid depressive disorders • Reactions to chronic stressors (e.g., fear of cancer recurrence, family/financial problems) • Side effects of regularly prescribed medications
Panic attacks present with paroxysmal acute anxiety	• Severe palpitations, diaphoresis and nausea. There is often a sense of great fear of a catastrophic event, described as a "feeling of impending doom." • Usually last for at least several minutes. The frequency is variable with multiple possible events in a single day.

Table 6.2   Etiology of Anxiety

Primary Psychiatric Disorders In the face of a cancer diagnosis or recurrence, exacerbations of these disorders may be anticipated. Patients with primary mood disorders and dementias also frequently experience symptoms of anxiety.	• Anxiety disorders are common in the general population. • These include generalized anxiety disorder (lifetime prevalence 5%). • panic disorder with/without agoraphobia (1-2%) • obsessive-compulsive disorder (2.5%) • post-traumatic stress disorder (PTSD) (8%)[4]

Cancer-Related: *Psychological* Anxiety can be interpreted as a reaction to threat.	• Anxiety increases in setting of:
	  • initial diagnosis;
	  • anticipation of check-ups;
	  • diagnostic studies that might detect recurrence;
	  • with advancing disease;
	  • news of poor prognosis;
	  • at the end of active treatment; or
	  • when surveillance intervals are increased.
	• Patients who are successfully treated may experience chronic anxiety related to fear of recurrence.
	• Patients who undergo genetic testing may also experience significant anxiety regarding their own health and that of their families.

(continued, next page)

Table 6.2   Etiology of Anxiety (continued)

Phobic reactions often present with anxiety that may escalate to full-blown panic	• Claustrophobic patients may have difficulty with procedures including magnetic resonance imaging scans and enforced long-term confinement in hospital (e.g., bone marrow transplant). • Needle phobia and "white coat syndrome" are especially problematic for some patients.
Conditioned responses	• Anticipatory nausea, often associated with anxiety. • Post-traumatic stress disorder in patients who survive cancer or who must undergo additional treatment.
Disease and Treatment-Related: May manifest at any time.[5] Consider increased likelihood of "organic" anxiety with increased acuity of medical illness.	• Congestive heart failure / pulmonary edema • Pulmonary embolism • Myocardial infarction • Hormone-secreting tumors (pheochromocytoma) • Seizure • Unrelieved pain
Disease complications: electrolyte abnormalities especially in patients with brain injury (i.e., dementia); delirium due to any cause; early indication of evolving sepsis; impending seizure.	• Hypercalcemia • Hyperthyroidism • Hypoglycemic • Hyponatremia • Hypoxia - initial consideration in any patient with pulmonary disease or anemia
Drugs Several drugs used in supportive oncology may be associated with anxiety. (Cf. Chapter 4, Table 4.1.)	• Anticholinergic, e.g. *benztropine*, *diphenhydramine* (Benadryl®) • Stimulants, e.g. *methylphenidate* (Ritalin®) • Sympathomimetics, e.g. *albuterol inhaler* • Steroids-mood lability and agitation • Immunosuppressants, e.g. *cyclosporine* • Drug withdrawal from benzodiazepines, alcohol, narcotics, barbituates • Older anti-emetics including *promethazine* (Phenergan®), *metoclopramide* (Reglan®), and *prochloroperazine* (Compazine®) can cause akathisia, a sense of severe internal anxiety and restlessness associated with motor agitation, i.e., pacing. • Anti-psychotics such as *haloperidol* (Haldol®), *risperidone* (Risperdol®), and *olanzapine* (Zyprexa®) can also cause akathisia. • Opioid analgesics and benzodiazepine anxiolytics may cause confusion or delirium in patients with cognitive impairment.

Evaluation

Patients experiencing anxiety should be thoroughly assessed for disease and treatment factors that may contribute to symptoms. The NCCN Distress Management Guidelines offer an algorithm (Figure 6.1).[6] The primary clinical team or a mental health specialist may search out contributing psychosocial factors. Several rating scales, including the State-Trait Anxiety Inventory, and the Hospital Anxiety and Depression Scale (pp. 7 - 8) may be used in cancer settings to help detect anxiety, though utility may be greater in research assessment of interventions than in clinical care.[13]

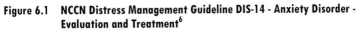

Figure 6.1   NCCN Distress Management Guideline DIS-14 - Anxiety Disorder - Evaluation and Treatment[6]

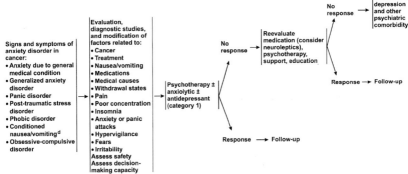

© *National Comprehensive Cancer Network, May 2005*

Interventions

Any medical or physical causes of anxiety should be identified and corrected if possible. If anxiety persists, then anti-anxiety medications may be useful.

Table 6.3   Anti-anxiety Medications*

Benzodiazepine (BZP) anxiolytics: Most often used for management of anxiety.[7] Generally safe, though respiratory suppression is possible in patients with compromised pulmonary function and those treated with central nervous system depressant agents. Patients with cognitive impairment of any type may become disinhibited or delirious when treated with BZPs. Potentially drugs of abuse, though that is usually not a problem in the oncology setting.

Short-acting drugs such as *lorazepam* (Ativan®) and *alprazolam* (Xanax®) have a rapid onset of action and are useful for intermittent acute anxiety or panic, and as pre-medications before procedures or tests. Preferred in more seriously ill patients. Longer acting drugs such as *diazepam* (Valium®) and *clonazepam* (Klonopin®) are useful for more persistent anxiety. Tolerance develops less rapidly with these drugs. Use cautiously in settings of hepatic impairment, critical illness, and in the elderly.

Table 6.3   Anti-anxiety Medications (continued)*

Antipsychotic drugs: Appropriate in patients vulnerable to adverse effects of BZPs (e.g., cognitive impairment, history of drug dependence).

Haloperidol (Haldol®), *olanzapine* (Zyprexa®), *quetiapine* (Seroquel®). Appropriate for anxiety in low doses, especially agitation or terror.

Opioid analgesics: Especially effective in management of anxiety in terminally ill patients, particularly when respiratory failure is a cause of anxiety.

morphine sulphate

Antidepressants: May have efficacy in the cancer setting for patients with preexisting anxiety disorders and in situations where anxiety is not expected to remit quickly. Antidepressants generally are not useful for "as needed" treatment of anxiety.

Especially selective serotonin reuptake inhibitors (SSRIs) i.e., *fluoxetine* (Prozac®), *sertraline* (Zoloft®), *paroxetine* (Paxil®), *citalopram* (Celexa®), *escitalopram* (Lexapro®). Also some others have become mainstays of treatment of chronic anxiety and panic disorders in the general population.[8]

* Cf. Chapter 4.

Table 6.4   Selected Drugs for Management of Anxiety in Cancer Patients*

Drug	Starting Dose	Maintenance Dose
Selective serotonin reuptake inhibitors		
escitalopram (Lexapro®)	10-20 mg	10-20 mg/day PO
fluoxetine (Prozac®)	10-20 mg qAM	20-60 mg/day PO
paroxetine (Paxil®)	20 mg/day qAM	20-60 mg/day PO
sertraline (Zoloft®)	25-50 mg qAM	50-150 mg/day PO
Benzodiazepines		
alprazolam (Xanax®)	0.25-1.0 mg	PO q 6-24h
clonazepam (Klonopin®)	0.5-2.0 mg	PO q 6-24h
diazepam (Valium®)	2-10 mg	PO/IV q 6-24h
lorazepam (Ativan®)	0.5-2.0 mg	PO/IM/IVP/IVPB q 4-12h

IM=intramuscular;   IVP = IV push;   IVPB = IV piggyback;   PO=oral

* Cf. Chapter 4.

Table 6.5   Psychotherapy and Behavioral Interventions for Anxiety

- Psychological interventions have well documented efficacy[9] to manage anxiety in cancer patients.
- Individual and group psychotherapy
- Behavioral interventions including relaxation, self-hypnosis, and guided imagery training.
- Many of these interventions require referral to a mental health professional or primary clinician trained in the appropriate treatment modality. This may or may not be practical, depending on resources and patient preferences.[3]
- In the primary oncology setting, supportive psychotherapy is almost universally appropriate and can be provided by most clinicians.[10]
- Decreases isolation and strengthens core coping skills
- Key components of supportive therapy: effective communication; patient education; involvement of family, institutional, and community support systems

Mood Disorders

Introduction

Clinicians will routinely encounter patients who appear "depressed".[11,12] Less often patients will present with elevated or expansive mood consistent with mania. Left untreated, these disorders are associated with treatment delays, complications, and increased costs. The differential diagnosis of depression-like presentations in cancer patients is lengthy. Accurate diagnosis can be difficult, but is important because treatment will vary depending on the actual cause of symptoms. Barriers to treatment include cultural factors and a presumption that depression is a natural consequence of cancer. Lack of agreed-upon screening instruments, lack of infrastructure for psychosocial support, and uncertainty about diagnosis and cost also add barriers.[13]

Table 6.6   DSM-IV-TR Criteria: Major Depressive Episode[14]

- Depressed mood
- Diminished interest or pleasure in activities
- Significant weight loss/gain or decrease/increase in appetite
- Insomnia or hypersomnia
- Fatigue or loss of energy
- Feelings of worthlessness or excessive guilt
- Diminished ability to think or concentrate, or indecisiveness
- Recurrent thoughts of death or suicidal ideation

Table 6.7   Syndromes of Mood

Major Depression Disorder: Patients who meet criteria for diagnosis of primary or secondary major depression (Table 6.6) will experience one or both of the hallmark emotional symptoms of depression (dysphoria, anhedonia) and at least five of the somatic symptoms. DSM-IV TR criteria also require the presence of vegetative and/or somatic symptoms, which, with psychological symptoms, must be present for at least two weeks and represent a distinct change from prior function.[12] A careful history is often needed to determine the etiology of these symptoms. Because the psychological or somatic cause of the symptoms may not be sorted with confidence, many researchers recommend that more emphasis be placed on psychological symptoms.

Psychological symptoms include *dysphoria* (sadness), lack of pleasure (*anhedonia),* *hopelessness*, and *feelings of guilt*. The first two of these, especially, are what most patients and clinicians consider to be "depression." Difficulty comes with consideration of the vegetative and somatic symptoms. Especially common in the experience of cancer and its treatment as well as depression are:
- changes in sleep;
- changes in appetite;
- changes in concentration; and
- loss of physical energy.

Adjustment disorders, e.g. the adjustment to the diagnosis of cancer, its course, and treatment

With the setbacks of cancer, patients may experience the **psychological symptoms** of depression with or without physical symptoms and are often very distressed. *Adjustment disorders* (also known as "minor depression" or "reactive depression") are the most common mood disorders diagnosed in cancer patients. The diagnosis requires that the patient experiences sadness or inability to take pleasure in life as a response to a stressor like cancer temporally related to the onset of symptoms, and that the symptoms are sufficiently severe that they cause impairment of social or occupational function. They may not meet criteria for major depression (Table 6.6) or secondary mood disorders because low mood is not persistent.

Primary or secondary mania

Psychological symptoms include elevated and expansive or irritable mood and rapid or pressured speech. Thought processes can seem illogical. Often demonstrate a decreased need for sleep, increased energy and impulsive or erratic behavior. Patients may speak of depressed mood when they are irritable.

Etiology

Assessment of mood disorders in cancer patients should include consideration of the patient's past history of anxiety and depressive disorders as well as specific reversible disease and treatment that can contribute to low mood.

Table 6.8   Etiology

Drugs	*Corticosteroids* especially in chronic use, may cause depressive syndromes and acutely may cause presentations consistent with mania. Central nervous system depressant medications, including *opioid analgesics, benzodiazepines, and barbiturates,* may cause depression in patients with idiosyncratic vulnerability or with cognitive impairment.
Antineoplastic drugs	Depressive syndromes may be encountered as side effects of *vinca alkyloids, L-asparaginase* and *procarbazine.* Of much greater concern are *biological response modifiers* including *interferon-alpha and interleukin-2 (IL-2).*[15] Interferon especially is associated with depression and may occasionally cause mania.
Metabolic abnormalities	Abnormalities of electrolytes (especially sodium), calcium, B-12 and folate, parathyroid function and especially thyroid function, can cause symptoms that are perceived and present as depression.
Tumor	A few primary malignancies have been associated with depression, such as occult carcinoma of the *pancreas, central nervous system lymphomas,* and *primary brain tumors.*
Unrelieved pain	Significant cause of depression in cancer patients Depression may also change a patient's perception of the meaning and severity of pain. Pain or the fear of unrelieved pain is a critical variable in requests for physician-assisted suicide.

Evaluation

Patients should be assessed when they or their families complain of depressive symptoms and when a mood disorder is suspected clinically. Rating scales are routinely used to screen for mood disorders. Some of the most popular include the Beck Depression Inventory (BDI or BDI-II),[16] and the Hospital Anxiety and Depression Scale (pp. 7 - 8). While these and other instruments can be very useful to identify patients who may be depressed, they are not sufficient to make a diagnosis of depression. They are not substitutes for a careful history and clinical examination of the patient. The examination should include assessment of the severity and duration of psychological and somatic symptoms, and their impact on the patient's quality of life and treatment of disease. Sometimes patients with cognitive impairment appear depressed but are suffering apathy or hypoactive delirium more than depression. Sometimes they have both depression and cognitive impairment.

Figure 6.2   NCCN Distress Management Guideline DIS-10, DIS-11 - Mood Disorder[17]

DIS-10

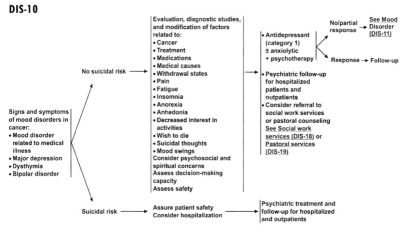

DIS-11 (linked from DIS-10)

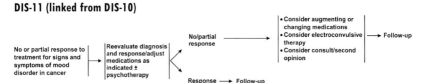

Table 6.9   Assessment of Suicide Potential*

- Patients with any type of mood disorder should be assessed for suicide risk.
- Conducted in an open, nonjudgmental manner- gives the patient "permission" to talk about thoughts that may be very frightening.
- Slightly indirect approach to the question of suicide risk may be helpful at first. The patient might be asked if he ever has thoughts that life is no longer worth living; if yes, does he have thoughts of ending his own life and if so, does he have a plan?
- It is fairly common for cancer patients to have *passive suicidal ideations* with no active desire to die, or plan.

Table 6.10 Risk Factors for Suicide*

• *active suicidal ideation* with desire/plan to die	• depression
• advanced disease	• social isolation
• uncontrolled pain	• physical and emotional exhaustion
• mild delirium	• alcohol or substance abuse
• past psychiatric history	• male gender[18]

Inteventions

Table 6.11 Management of Suicide Threat*

- Safety of patients at risk for suicide must be secured.
- Do not leave alone until they can be evaluated and started in treatment.
- May need to pursue voluntary or involuntary admission to hospital.
- Any disease and treatment related factors (especially pain) that may be contributing to the presenting mood disorder should be addressed.

Table 6.12 Psychotherapy for Mood Disorders

- Supportive psychotherapy in patients with major and minor depression is almost universally appropriate as one element of treatment.
- Goal: decrease perception of isolation, and bolster coping skills.
- Support can be provided by members of the primary team and also by allied health professionals including social workers and chaplains.
- More formal and structured psychotherapy may be appropriate on a case-by-case basis. This involves referral to a mental health professional of any discipline with appropriate training.

* Cf. Chapter 3.

Table 6.13 Medication Management

Antidepressants and mood stabilizers: Choice of antidepressant usually is based on side effect profile.

- No antidepressant formulations allow parenteral administration.
- The use of antidepressants is a matter of clinical judgment.
- Patients who meet criteria for major depression should be treated.
- Patients with severe adjustment disorders or who do not meet full criteria for depression may also benefit from antidepressant therapy.
- Almost all of the antidepressants available in general clinical practice can be used in cancer patients.[19]
- *Selective serotonin reuptake inhibitor (SSRI)* antidepressants *(citalopram, fluoxetine, escitalopram, paroxetine, sertraline)* and the newer combination agents *(bupropion, duloxetine, venlafaxine, mirtazapine)* are used most frequently in oncology because of their safety and generally favorable side effect profiles. (Cf. Table 6.14 and Chapter 4, Table 4.2.)
- *Tricyclic antidepressants* (TCAs) are potentially problematic because of anticholinergic and anti-alpha-adrenergic effects. However, they are inexpensive and can be useful in patients with co-morbid neuropathic pain syndromes. (Cf. Table 6.14 and Chapter 4, Table 4.3.)
- They take anywhere from 2-4 weeks to take effect.
- Patients should be monitored for side effects and response of symptoms.
- Seriously ill and elderly patients should be started at low doses, with cautious dose escalation if the drug is tolerated.
- Continue for 4-6 months of sustained response before considering discontinuation.
- Cancer patients with preexisting bipolar mood disorder ideally should be maintained on mood stabilizers (i.e., *lithium, valproic acid)* and antipsychotic medications. Dehydration associated with treatment-associated vomiting and diarrhea can affect lithium levels, which should be monitored closely during active treatment.
- *Monoamine oxidase inhibitor* antidepressants (MAOIs) are very difficult to use in this setting because of drug-drug and drug-food interactions and should be avoided.

(continued, next page)

Table 6.13 Medication Management (continued)

Psychostimulants	• Stimulants like *d-amphetamine, modafinil,* and *methylphenidate* are used in depressed medically ill patients. • Can be very beneficial in treatment of associated fatigue, mild cognitive impairment, and anorexia, especially in advanced and end-stage disease settings.[20] • More rapid effect than standard antidepressants • Generally well tolerated but can have adverse effects on blood pressure
Antipsychotic drugs	• *Steroid-induced mania* will usually respond to decrease of steroid doses. • In some cases this is not feasible and the patient will require treatment with an antipsychotic drug such as *olanzapine.* (Cf. Chapter 4, Table 4.6.)

Table 6.14 Selected Antidepressants Used in Cancer Patients*

Drug	Starting Dose	Maint. Dose	Comments
Selective serotonin reuptake inhibitors			
citalopram (Celexa®)	10 mg/day	20 - 40 mg/day	Soltabs new in 2006
escitalopram (Lexapro®)	5 - 10 mg/day	10 - 20 mg/day	Possible nausea, sexual dysfunction
fluoxetine (Prozac®)	10 - 20 mg/day	20 - 60 mg/day	Long half-life; possible nausea, sexual dysfunction
paroxetine (Paxil®)	20 mg/day	20 - 60 mg/day	Possible nausea, sedation
sertraline (Zoloft®)	25 - 50 mg/day	50 - 150 mg/day	Possible nausea
Tricyclic antidepressants			
amitriptyline (Elavil®)	25 - 50 mg qhs	50-200 mg/day	Maximal sedation; anticholinergic effects; useful for neuropathic pain
desipramine (Norpramin®)	25 - 50 mg/day	50-200 mg/day	Modest sedation; anticholinergic effects; useful for neuropathic pain
nortriptyline (Pamelor®)	25 - 50 mg qhs	50-200 mg/day	Moderate sedation; useful for neuropathic pain

* Cf. Chapter 4.

(continued, next page)

Table 6.14 Selected Antidepressants Used in Cancer Patients (continued)*

Other agents

bupropion (Wellbutrin®)	75 mg/day	150 mg/day tid or XR; 300 mg XL	Activating; no reports of sexual dysfunction; risk of seizures in predisposed patients
duloxetine (Cymbalta®)	20 - 40 mg/day	60 mg/day	Possible nausea, dry mouth; may be useful for neuropathic pain
methylphenidate (Ritalin®)	5 mg (2.5 mg qAM, noon)	10 - 60 mg/day	Activating; rapid effect possible; monitor blood pressure
mirtazapine (Remeron®)	15 mg qhs	15 - 45 mg qhs	Sedating, variable appetite-stimulant, antiemetic effects
venlafaxine (Effexor®)	18.75 - 37.5 mg/day	75 - 225 mg/day	XR is daily; possible nausea; may be useful for neuropathic pain, hot flashes

Cognitive Disorders

Introduction

Cognitive disorders are the second most common psychiatric disorders in oncology. Prevalence of delirium and dementia will increase as the general population ages and patients live longer with cancer. Delirium, also called acute confusional state or encephalopathy, contributes to increased morbidity and mortality, treatment costs, and stress in caregivers. Delirium is more prevalent among the old, critical care patients, and those with end stage disease.[21,22,23] Dementia also predisposes to delirium. Complicating assessment and treatment are: imprecise nomenclature for cognitive deficits; sometimes subtle, inconsistent, and overlapping signs and symptoms; and multiple etiologies.

Delirium

Table 6.15 Clinical Features of Delirium[22,24]

- Acute onset
- Confusion, disorientation, impaired reality testing
- Inability to pay attention (distractibility)
- Psychomotor agitation or retardation
- Illusions (misperceptions) and hallucinations (usually visual)
- Diurnal variation (worse at night, early AM)
- Sleep-wake cycle disruption
- Lucid intervals
- Autonomic dysfunction
- Fear and anxiety
- Delusions, especially with paranoid themes

Table 6.16 Risk Factors for Delirium

· Advanced age	· Sensory deprivation (hearing or vision loss) [25]
· Acuity of illness	· End organ damage
· History of cognitive impairment	· History of alcoholism
· Medication	

Table 6.17 Common Causes of Delirium

Infection	• Fever
Metabolic disturbance	• Hypoxia • Hypercapnia • Hyperglycemia • Hypo- or hyper-glycemia • Electrolyte disturbance • Impaired liver function • Impaired kidney function
Drugs	• Central nervous system depressants • Corticosteroids • Sympathomimetics • Anticholinergic medications • Opioid analgesics • Benzodiazepine sedative-hypnotics • Alcohol or drug intoxication
Drug withdrawal	• Especially alcohol and benzodiazapines
Cancer Therapies	• Chemotherapy agents (ifosfamide, methotrexate, cytosine arabinoside) [26,27] • Biotherapy agents, e.g. interleukin-2 (IL-2), interferon-alpha [28] • Brain radiation (early, late-delayed syndromes) • Supportive therapy agents (opioids, benzodiazepines)
Seizure-related	• Post-ictal • Complex partial status epilepticus
Disease-related	• Unrelieved pain • Direct and indirect effects of primary brain tumors • Central nervous system metastasis • Paraneoplastic syndromes (rarely) • Terminal stages of disease-heralds end of the disease trajectory [29]

Figure 6.3 NCCN Distress Management Guidelines DIS-9 - Delirium[30]

EVALUATION/TREATMENT/FOLLOW-UP

© National Comprehensive Cancer Network, May 2005

Table 6.18 Evaluation of the Delirious Patient[31]

- History and chart review
- Attention to medications administered and discontinued
- Clinical interview and mental status examination
- Physical examination; attention to neurological status
- Laboratory assessment: complete blood count with differential and platelets, electrolytes, glucose, creatinine, BUN, O_2 saturation/arterial blood gasses, calcium, magnesium, albumin, liver function tests, thyroid function tests, RPR
- Chest x-ray, EKG,
- Urine, blood cultures, cerebral spinal fluid studies, if indicated
- Serum/urine drug and alcohol screens
- As indicated: B12 and folate levels, serum drug levels, EEG, brain CT/MRI
- Rating scales: Delirium Rating Scale, the Memorial Delirium Assessment Scale (cf. Chapter 2), and the Confusion Assessment Method[32]

Table 6.19 Selected Medications for Management of Delirium[31,33,*]

Antipsychotics	• haloperidol[†] (Haldol®) 0.5 - 5 mg q 30 min - 12h PO, IM, IV
	• chlorpromazine[†] (Thorazine®) 25 - 100 mg q 4 - 12h PO, IM, IV
	• risperidone (Risperdol®) 0.5 - 2 mg q 12h PO
	• olanzapine (Zyprexa®) 2.5 - 5 mg q 12 - 24h PO, IM[34]
	• quetiapine (Seroquel®) 12.5 - 50 mg q 12h PO
Benzodiazepines	• lorazepam[†] (Ativan®) 0.5 - 2 mg q 1 - 4h PO, IM, IV
	• midazolam[†] (Versed®) 0.003 mg/kg/h titrate to effect IV (per anesthesiologist)

[†] *may be administered by continuous infusion, usually in the intensive care setting.*

* Cf. Chapter 4.   (continued, next page)

Table 6.19 Selected Medications for Management of Delirium (continued)

Anesthetics	• propofol[†] (Diprivan®) 0.5 mg/kg/hr titrate to effect IV
Alpha Agonists	• dexmedetomidine (Precedex®) 1 mcg/kg over 10 min followed by continuous infusion 0.2-0.7 mcg/kg/hr • Intensive care setting: *propofol* and *dexmedetomadine* provide rapid sedation with prompt resolution of effect when discontinued.[35] These foster sedation but do not improve cognition.

[†] *may be administered by continuous infusion, usually in the intensive care setting.*

Table 6.20 Delirium - Managing Safety and Environment

Prevent accidental self-harm	• Falls • Pulled IV lines • Pulled catheters
Close observation	• Family • Nurse • Sitter • Physical restraints if necessary
Physical agitation and physiological instability	• Admit to intensive care setting
Physical environment	• Adequate, but not excessive, sensory stimulation • Minimize disruption of sleep-wake cycle • Lights on during day • Avoid long periods of daytime sleep • Frequent reorientation • Address sensory deficits (eyeglasses, hearing aids) • Night: low-level background light and sound (music or television) maintained • Family presence- comforting
Caregiver concerns- frightened, embarrassed, ashamed, highly stressed, grief-stricken	• Communicate and educate about delirium and how it will be managed. • Family members should be encouraged to take breaks. May be better if distressed family members do not stay with the patient, especially overnight. • One-to-one monitoring by professional patient aides helps ensure patient safety and allows family members to get needed rest.[36]

Dementia

Table 6.21 General Diagnostic Criteria for Dementia[4]

- Memory impairment (impaired ability to learn new information or to recall previously learned information)
- One (or more) of the following cognitive disturbances
  - aphasia (language disturbance)
  - apraxia (impaired ability to carry out motor activities despite intact motor function)
  - agnosia (failure to recognize or identify objects despite intact sensory function)
  - disturbance in executive functioning (i.e., planning, organizing, sequencing, abstracting)

Table 6.22 Etiology of Apparent Dementia

Cancer/Treatment-related	• Metastatic brain tumor • Systemic cancer (small cell lung cancer) • Leptomeningeal carcinomatosis • Paraneoplastic syndrome • Disease progression and complications • Nutritional deficiencies (cobalamin, niacin) • Small or large brain infarcts • Anemia
Hypoactive delirium	• Easily confused with dementia. (Patient is quietly impaired, but this is fluctuating and reversible.)
Severe depression	• Thinking is slow. Cognitive impairment concerns the patient, but formal cognition less impaired.
Antineoplastic Therapies	• Antimetabolites, e.g. methotrexate, ifosphamide, cytosine arabinoside • Biological response modifiers, e.g. interferon, interleukin-2 (IL-2) • Brain radiation (late-delayed radiation toxicity)[37,38]
Supportive Care Drugs	• Central nervous system (CNS) depressants (opioid analgesics, benzodiazepine anxiolytics and hypnotics, anticonvulsants, and some antidepressants) may cause temporary cognitive impairment.

Figure 6.4   NCCN Distress Management Guidelines DIS-7, DIS-8 - Dementia[39]

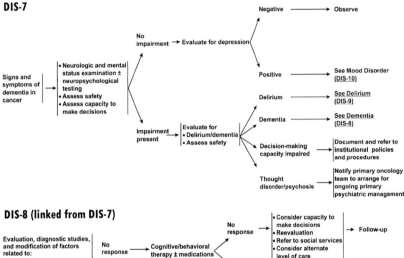

© National Comprehensive Cancer Network, May 2005

Table 6.23 Evaluation for Dementia

Mental status and physical examination	• Emphasizes attention, concentration and memory function, language, executive function, and judgment[40] • Standardized screening instruments are recommended: Mini-Mental State Examination (MMSE) is most frequently used (pp. 9 - 11).[41] • Physical examination emphasizes neurological function.
Laboratory, imaging, and neuropsychological tests	• Electrolytes, renal and hepatic function, endocrine function, and nutritional status (e.g., albumin, serum B12 and folate levels). • Neuroimaging should be used if CNS disease (tumor, cerebrovascular accident) is suspected. • Neuropsychological testing: extremely useful in assessment of subtle deficits, executive function, differential diagnosis, treatment planning and treatment response, and in some cases, rehabilitation.

(continued, next page)

Table 6.23 Evaluation for Dementia (continued)

Capacity and safety	• Determine ability to make selected decisions and to understand consequences. • Patient needs adequate supervision. • Patient may have significant difficulties with informed consent process.

Table 6.24 Management of Dementia

Pharmacotherapy	• Antidepressants • Antipsychotics • Benzodiazepine anxiolytics- use cautiously, if at all • Psychostimulants[42,43]
Behavior	• Use cognitive cues, reorientation, and maintenance of consistent environments. • Some patients may benefit from cognitive rehabilitation.
Caregivers	• Assessed regarding their abilities to cope with the demands involved in the care of a cognitively impaired patient • Caregiver support groups, and individual and family therapy • Referral to allied mental health specialists including psychiatrists, psychologists, and social workers if required care is beyond the capacity of the primary clinical service.

Substance Abuse

Introduction

For patients with pain, the stigma of a remote or current history of drug abuse can complicate management of cancer and its psychosocial dimension. In order to manage cancer pain optimally, the staff must understand the complex interface between drug abuse and therapeutic use of drugs that can be abused. Approximately one-third of the population in the United States has used illicit drugs and an estimated 6-15% have a substance use disorder of some type.[44,45,46] Only when the addiction problems and the patient's special needs are recognized can these patients be successfully treated.[47]

Table 6.25 Substance Abuse Definitions

- Traditional definitions of addiction that include concepts of physical dependence or tolerance cannot be the model terminology for medically ill populations who receive drugs for legitimate medical purposes that can be abused.
- A chronic substance abuse disorder is characterized by "the compulsive use of a substance resulting in physical, psychological or social harm to the user and continued use despite that harm."[48]
- Loss of control over drug use, compulsive drug use, and continued use despite harm are key features.
- The concept of "aberrant drug-related behavior" is a useful first step to operationalize the definitions of abuse and addiction, and to recognize the broad range of behaviors that may be considered problematic by prescribers.
- If drug-taking behavior in a medical patient can be characterized as aberrant, a differential diagnosis for this behavior can be explored.

Table 6.26 Differential Diagnosis of Aberrant Drug-taking Attitudes & Behaviors

Addiction	"Use despite harm" concept
Pseudoaddiction	Inadequate analgesia leading to acting out (ie, self-medicating, using alcohol or street drugs, doctor shopping, etc.) to treat pain
Other Psychiatric Diagnoses: • Encephalopathy • Borderline personality disorder • Depression • Anxiety	Many times, psychiatric illness or complications are reported as untreated pain. These symptoms may best be considered as "suffering" that adds to the pain complaints.
Criminal Intent	Small subset of criminals who are out solely for diversion and profit

Substance Abuse Screening and Evaluation

In assessing the differential diagnosis for drug-related behavior, it is useful to consider the degree of aberrancy. The less aberrant behaviors (such as aggressively complaining about the need for medications) are more likely to reflect untreated distress of some type, rather than addiction-related concerns. The more aberrant behaviors (such as injection of an oral formulation) are more likely to reflect true addiction.

By making a distinction between patients with no histories of substance abuse and those who are prior addicts, as well as all the gradations between, chronic pain management can be tailored to the patient. To this end, we offer an oversimplified three-level conceptualization of prototypical patients and the amount of follow-up necessary for each. While these are caricatures, they should be used to create mental prototypes as we see and assess chronic pain patients (Table 6.27).

Table 6.27 Prototypical Patients - Requirements for Pain Management

"Nice Little Old Lady" (uncomplicated patient)	• Minimal structure required due to lack of comorbid psychiatric problems and lack of connection to drug subculture • Routine medical management is generally sufficient. • Suggested practice: 30-day supply of medications with liberal rescue dose policy • Monthly follow-ups
"The Chemical Coper"	• Behavior resembles that of addicts with a central focus on obtaining drugs. • Needs structure, psychiatric input, and drug treatments that decentralize the pain medication from their coping • Reduce meaning of medications; undo conditioning; undo socialization around the drug. • Best accomplished via psychotherapy focused on pain
"Addicted Patient" • Active abuser • Patient in drug-free recovery • Patient in methadone maintenance	• Requires the most structure including frequent visits • Give patient a limited supply of medications. • Drug choices should be tailored for long-acting opioids with little street value. • Rescues offered judiciously • Implement use of urine toxicology screening and follow-up on results. • Require patient to be in active recovery programs or psychotherapy.

Table 6.28 Domains of Pain Management Outcome: The 4 As[49]

Outcome Area	Explanation
Analgesia	• Actual amount of nociceptive relief experienced by the chosen opioid therapy • Most obvious "A" - should not be considered the only important part of opioid therapy
Activities of Daily Living	• Whether or not the patient on opioid therapy has become more active in their life as a result of opioid therapy • Domains of interest include physical, social, emotional, and family functioning as well as improved sleep.
Adverse Side Effects	• Whether or not opioid therapy chosen has intolerable side effects for the patient • Typical adverse effects include constipation, nausea, sedation, and mental clouding.
Aberrant Drug Related Behaviors	These are "ambiguous non-compliance behaviors." In essence, whether or not the patient is engaging in socially undesirable behaviors with their opioid therapy that may or may not be indicative of addiction. Problem behaviors include: • self-escalating doses; • hoarding medications; • seeking out multiple providers for prescriptions, • prescription forgery; and • stealing prescription drugs.

Table 6.29 Two Key Rules of Good Opioid Pain Treatment

- The clinician must maintain an accepting and thoughtful attitude directed toward self-reports of pain.
- Prudent drug selection and the decision to use an opioid must be followed by titration of the dose to maintain a balance between effective analgesia and opioid side effects.

Figure 6.6   NCCN Distress Management Guidelines DIS-15, DIS-16 - Substance Abuse[50]

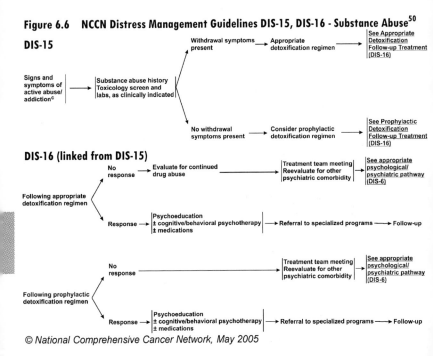

© *National Comprehensive Cancer Network, May 2005*

Interventions

Table 6.30 Substance Abuse Treatments

- Consider the unique pharmacological needs of addicts and then add the additional structures for recovery and psychosocial support to maximize the likelihood of a good outcome. These are complex patients who have two distinct diseases, substance abuse and cancer. Treatment with the assumption that anti-cancer treatment is most important and will "take care" of the second ailment of substance abuse is a common mistake that results in additional suffering for the patient.
- Connect with the patient, form a therapeutic bond, so that more reliable self-reports about drug use and trust can be maintained by both parties.
- Get the patients to articulate what help they most need.   (continued, next page)

Table 6.30 Treatments for Substance Abuse (continued)

• Pain reports should be followed by non-judgmental, interested, and concerned assessment that recognizes the cry of distress.
• Drug addicts have often been described as alexithymic and many are unable to label distress more precisely than globally good or bad. It is often this trait that leads to global distress in the face of the negative emotions associated with pain and chronic illness.[51]
• Drug selection is often limited to sustained-release delivery to avoid supporting compulsive pill popping and/or use of opioids in the service of chemical coping.[47]
• Use a drug with a relatively lower street value for patients who are in recovery but who still maintain contact with the addiction subculture.
• The dose is titrated and continued for effect or toxicity, bearing in mind that addicts will often be highly tolerant and require very large doses of opioids for pain control.
• Urine screening can be a very useful tool for the practicing clinician, both to diagnose abuse problems and to monitor patients with an established history of abuse. Sometimes the test would document whether the patient is taking what has been prescribed; sometimes the test would say if the patient is taking what has not been prescribed.

Personality Disorders
Introduction
In the Diagnostic and Statistical Manual for Mental Disorders, 4th Edition (DSM-IV),[52] personality disorders are placed into 3 clusters: the odd or eccentric; the avoidant and paranoid; and the impulsive/self-centered. Patients with personality disorders who face the anxiety and discomfort associated with medical treatment can have difficulties with medical caregivers, distort reality for emotional protection, or exhibit outright aggression and self-destructiveness.[53]

Table 6.31 Key Attributes of Personality Disorder

• A consistent pattern of behaviors that deviates markedly from the expectations of the individual's culture
• Stable over time
• Pervasive and inflexible
• Has onset in adolescence or early adulthood
• Thought to be poor coping or defense mechanisms used to buffer residual high stress that has not been overcome
• Leads to distrust or impairment

Table 6.32 Types of Personality Disorders & their Key Components[54,55]

Paranoid	• Suspicious of others • Perceives attacks by others quickly • Categorizes people as an enemy or friend • Rarely confides in others • Unforgiving
Schizoid	• Flat affect • Tends to be solitary in nature • Indifferent to criticism and praise • Marked absence of close friends or relationships
Schizotypal	• Has magical thinking or odd beliefs • Exhibits anxiety in social situations • Paranoid ideation • Experiences unusual perceptions
Antisocial	• Lacks conformity to laws • Ignores obligations • Impulsive • Irritable and aggressive
Borderline	• Fears of abandonment • Suicidal behavior • Mood instability • Chronic feelings of emptiness
Histrionic	• Easily influenced • Rapidly shifting emotions • Theatrical emotions • Provocative or sexual behavior
Narcissistic	• Belief in being "special" • Lacks empathy • Arrogant • Sense of entitlement
Avoidant	• Self view as inferior • Inhibited in new relationships • Tries to avoid embarrassment • Fear of rejection in social situations

(continued, next page)

Table 6.32 Types of Personality Disorders & their Key Components (continued)

Dependent	• Fears of being left alone • Lack of self-confidence • Requires reassurance when making decisions • Unlikely to express disagreement for fear of rejection
Obsessive-Compulsive	• Preoccupied with details • Tendency for perfectionism • Inflexible and stubborn • Unable to discard worthless objects
Personality Disorder NOS	• Reserved for disorders that do not fit any of the other categories • Can also describe people who exhibit features of several personality disorders without meeting full criteria for any one disorder

Table 6.33 Personality Disorder Screening and Evaluation

Taking a Psychological History	• Be straightforward in assessing a taboo subject. • Those with past history of psychological distress or personality disorders are more likely to suffer from both in the future. • Personaility Disorders are difficult to diagnose. • Significant comorbidity exists among personality disorders. • Comorbidity leads to difficulty in identifying a primary personality diagnosis. • Axis I disorders will complicate the identification of personality disorders.[56,57]
The physician's perspective	• The clinician with the personality-disordered patient does not need to make the diagnosis to be successful, but he or she must respond to the behavior. • Avoid stereotyping patients. • Be aware of your own feelings towards your patients, especially those who cause you to have emotional reactions.
Make a referral to a Mental Health Provider: social worker, psychologist, or psychiatrist, depending on what is available in your community/organization.*	• Cancer patients utilize mental health professionals more often than the general public (7.2% v 5.7%).[58] • When a patient is challenging the resources of the physician and staff, it is a wise decision to enroll the aid of a Mental Health Provider.

* It is always useful to establish a relationship in your practice with Mental Health Providers. They should have an understanding and respect for the challenges of dealing with cancer patients who also have a comorbid personality disorder. Frequent feedback and discussion of the patient's status is helpful to all involved.

Figure 6.7   NCCN Distress Management Guidelines DIS-17 - Personality Disorder[59]

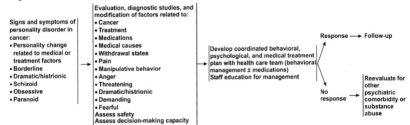

© *National Comprehensive Cancer Network, May 2005*

Interventions

Table 6.34 Personality Disorder Treatments

Management of the psychiatric disorder	• That therapist will work on limit setting and behavior modification with patient and staff. • The physician and other healthcare staff need to remember the frame of treatment and not be dragged into covering too many psychosocial issues and crises. • At times, it might be necessary to develop a signed agreement with the patient about this frame of treatment and what limits are in place with various members of the treating team.
Psychopharmacology	While personality disorder is best treated with psychotherapy and minimization of patient opportunity to manipulate care, there is a limited role for pharmacotherapy for specific issues. Consider the following to address features that might accompany the personality disorder: • mood disorders (antidepressants or lithium); • psychotic symptoms (antipsychotics); • anxiety symptoms (anxiolytics or antipsychotics); and • possible expanded role for atypical antipsychotics.
Management of the impact of the patient's behavior on staff behavior	• Management of staff issues is critical. • Staff meetings with all those involved in the patient's care can be very helpful. • New responses to the patient's behaviors can be planned. • Maintain teamwork to manage difficult patients. • Avoiding staff splitting (ie, do not let the patient "tell stories" about other staff members in order to create staff tension and distrust amongst the healthcare team).

Brief Intervention - The FRAMES Technique

Physicians can often feel unnerved by dealing with difficult patients who have personality disorders. They may begin to avoid interactions with the patients and feel that they always end in confrontations. The following FRAMES technique is a handy way to structure contacts with these patients while delivering needed information in a structured way.

Table 6.35 The FRAMES Technique

Feedback	• Deliver information. • Make observations. • Be non-judgmental, non-blaming. • Identify *behaviors* indicative of abuse and addiction; use checklists.

Responsibility	• Remind the patient that they have a role in their treatment that may be hampered by their behavior: "I am concerned that you have two problems — your cancer and possibly a problem dealing with stress." (or substance abuse/depression/anxiety...)
	• Treatment for the problem is the patient's responsibility:
	  • "Think about what I have said."
	  • "Observe your behaviors."
	  • "Make a decision about your treatment."

Advice	• Offer advice from the stance of expert medical opinion instead of reward/punishment or referrent authority. • Use a neutral tone: "You could take your MRI to another physician and get more drugs, but I do not advise this."
Menu	• Offer multiple treatment choices (and identify whether there are *multiple problems*). • Will assist with finding the best option for them. • "You may not be ready now, but I will be here for you if you change your mind at some point in the future."
Empathy	• "I know that you have been through a lot." • Patients do not consciously choose to become addicted, adopt the sick role, become depressed, etc. • Use understanding, compassion, insight. • Without blame, empathy becomes easier.
Self-Efficacy	• "I know this is very hard but I also know that you can do this." • Repeat any strengths patient has revealed by *report* and by *your observations*. • Ends intervention on a positive note. • Re-emphasize that responsibility belongs to the patient.

The Angry Patient:

It is very common for patients with personality disorders to exhibit their frustrations and to take their anger out on staff and other healthcare team members. The following tips are useful to prevent escalation of the patient's outbursts and escalation of staff anger and frustration. Ultimately, the goal is to help the patients to regain control and to learn to cope better with the issues that face them.

Table 6.36 Management of the Angry Patient

- Do not personalize.
- Listen to their perspective.
- Acknowledge their view.
- Check for accuracy, listen for feelings, listen for the underlying problem.
- Empathize.
- Reframe.
- Focus on different interpretations rather than "truth" (ie, we see things differently).
- Focus on responsibility rather than blame.
- Focus on intentions and outcomes rather than accusations.
- Be clear about your decisions.
- Share your perspective — with clarity.
- Ask for feedback.
- Problem solve.
- Remember, not everyone will be happy.
- Retreat (find a colleague if necessary).
- Reevaluate.
- Reapproach.
- Make another appointment if necessary.

References

Anxiety Disorders

1. Stark D, Kiely M, Smith A, Velikova G, House A & Selby P (2002). Anxiety disorders in cancer patients: Their nature, associations, and relation to quality of life. *Journal of Clinical Oncology*, 20, 3137-3148.

2. Noyes R, Holt CS & Massie MJ (1998). Anxiety disorders. In MJ Massie (Ed.), Psychiatric disorders. In JC Holland (Ed.), *Psycho-oncology* (pp. 548-563). New York: Oxford University Press.

3. Stark DP & House A (2000). Anxiety in cancer patients. *British Journal of Cancer*, 83, 1261-1267.

4. American Psychiatric Association. (1994). *Diagnostic and statistical manual of mental disorders* (4th ed.). Washington, DC: Author.

5. Goldberg MD & Posner DA (2000). Anxiety in the medically ill. In A Stoudemire, BS Fogel & DB Greenberg (Eds.), *Psychiatric care of the medical patient* (pp. 165-180). New York: Oxford University Press.

6. Anxiety Disorder (DIS-14). Reproduced with permission from the NCCN 1.2005 Distress Management, The Complete Library of NCCN Clinical Practice Guidelines in Oncology [CD-Rom]. Jenkintown, Pennsylvania: ©National Comprehensive Cancer Network, May 2005. To view the most recent and complete version of the guidelines, go online to www.nccn.org.*

7. Stiefel F, Berney A & Mazzocato C (1999). Psychopharmacology in supportive care in cancer: A review for the clinician. I. Benzodiazepines. *Supportive Care in Cancer, 7*, 379-385.

8. Fricchione G (2004). Clinical practice. Generalized anxiety disorder. *New England Journal of Medicine, 351*, 675-682.

9. Redd WH, Montgomery GH & DuHamel KN (2001). Behavioral intervention for cancer treatment side effects. *Journal of the National Cancer Institute, 93*, 810-823.

10. Epstein SA & Hicks D (2005). Anxiety disorders. In JL Levenson (Ed.), *The American psychiatric publishing textbook of psychosomatic medicine* (pp. 251-270). Washington, DC: American Psychiatric Publishing, Inc.

Mood Disorders

11. Newport DJ & Nemeroff CB (1998). Assessment and treatment of depression in the cancer patient. *Journal of Psychosomatic Research, 45*, 215-237.

12. Chochinov HM (2001). Depression in cancer patients. *Lancet Oncology, 2*, 499-505.

13. Greenberg DB (2004). Barriers to the treatment of depression in cancer patients. *Journal of the National Cancer Institute. Monographs, (32)*, 127-135.

14. American Psychiatric Association. (1994). *Diagnostic and statistical manual of mental disorders* (4th ed.). Washington, DC: Author

15. Capuron L, Ravaud A & Dantzer R (2000). Early depressive symptoms in cancer patients receiving interleukin 2 and/or interferon alfa-2b therapy. *Journal of Clinical Oncology, 18*, 2143-2151.

16. Beck, AT, Steer, RA, Brown GK (1996). *Beck Depression Inventory®—II (BDI®–II)*. San Antonio, Texas: Boston: Psychological Corporation; Harcourt Brace.

17. Mood Disorders (DIS-10, -11). Reproduced with permission from the *NCCN 1.2005 Distress Management, The Complete Library of NCCN Clinical Practice Guidelines in Oncology [CD-Rom]*. Jenkintown, Pennsylvania: ©National Comprehensive Cancer Network, May 2005. To view the most recent and complete version of the guidelines, go online to www.nccn.org.*

18. Massie MJ & Greenberg DB (2005). Oncology. In JL Levenson (Ed.), *The American psychiatric publishing textbook of psychosomatic medicine* (pp. 517-534). Washington, DC: American Psychiatric Publishing, Inc.

19. Berney A, Stiefel F, Mazzocato C & Buclin T (2000). Psychopharmacology in supportive care of cancer: A review for the clinician. III. Antidepressants. *Supportive Care in Cancer, 8*, 278-286.

20. Homsi J, Nelson KA, Sarhill N, Rybicki L, LeGrand SB, Davis MP, et al. (2000). A phase II study of methylphenidate for depression in advanced cancer. *American Journal of Hospice & Palliative Care, 18*, 403-407.

Cognitive Disorders

21. Lawlor PG & Bruera ED (2002). Delirium in patients with advanced cancer. *Hematology/Oncology Clinics of North America, 16*, 701-714.

22. Lipowski ZJ (1990). *Delirium: Acute confusional states.* New York: Oxford University Press.

23. Massie MJ, Holland J & Glass E (1983). Delirium in terminally ill cancer patients. *American Journal of Psychiatry, 140*, 1048-1050.

24. American Psychiatric Association. (1994). *Diagnostic and statistical manual of mental disorders* (4th ed.). Washington, DC: Author

25. Liptzin B (2000). Clinical diagnosis and management of delirium. In A Stoudemire, BS Fogel & DB Greenberg (Eds.), *Psychiatric Care of the Medical Patient* (2nd ed., pp. 581-596). New York: Oxford University Press.

26. Brown TM (2000). Drug-induced delirium. *Seminars in Clinical Neuropsychiatry, 5*, 113-124.

27. Breitbart W & Cohen KR (1998). Delirium. In MJ Massie (Ed.), Psychiatric disorders. In JC Holland (Ed.), *Psycho-Oncology* (pp.564-575). New York: Oxford University Press.

28. Meyers CA & Valentine AD (1995). Neurological and psychiatric adverse effects of immunological therapy. *CNS Drugs, 3*, 56-68.

29. Breitbart W & Cohen K (2000). Delirium in the terminally ill. In HM Chochinov & W Breitbart (Eds.), *Handbook of Psychiatry in Palliative Medicine* (pp. 75-90). New York: Oxford University Press.

30. Delirium and Dementia (DIS -9). Reproduced with permission from the *NCCN 1.2005 Distress Management, The Complete Library of NCCN Clinical Practice Guidelines in Oncology [CD-Rom].* Jenkintown, Pennsylvania: ©National Comprehensive Cancer Network, May 2005. To view the most recent and complete version of the guidelines, go online to www.nccn.org.*

31. Valentine AD & Bickham J (2005). Delirium and Substance Withdrawal. In A Shaw, BJ Riedel, AW Burton, AI Fields & TJ Feeley (Eds.), *Acute Care of the Cancer Patient* (pp 545-557). New York: Marcel Dekker.

32. Trzepacz PT (1994). A review of delirium assessment instruments. *General Hospital Psychiatry, 16,* 397-405.

33. Bruera E, Franco JJ, Maltoni M, Watanabe S & Suarez-Almazor M (1995). Changing pattern of agitated impaired mental status in patients with advanced cancer: Association with cognitive monitoring, hydration, and opioid rotation. *Journal of Pain and Symptom Management, 1,* 287-291.

34. Breitbart W, Tremblay A & Gibson C (2002). An open trial of olanzapine for the treatment of delirium in hospitalized cancer patients. *Psychosomatics, 43,* 175-182.

35. Breitbart W, Gibson C & Tremblay A (2002). The delirium experience: Delirium recall and delirium-related distress in hospitalized patients with cancer, their spouses/caregivers, and their nurses. *Psychosomatics, 43,* 183-194.

36. Liptzin B & Levkoff SE (1992). An empirical study of delirium subtypes. *British Journal of Psychiatry, 161,* 843-845.

37. Verstappen CC, Heimans JJ, Hoekman K & Postma TJ (2003). Neurotoxic complications of chemotherapy in patients with cancer: Clinical signs and optimal management. *Drugs, 63,* 1549-1563.

38. New P (2001). Radiation injury to the nervous system. *Current Opinion in Neurology, 14,* 725-734.

39. Delirium and Dementia (DIS-7, -8). Reproduced with permission from the *NCCN 1.2005 Distress Management, The Complete Library of NCCN Clinical Practice Guidelines in Oncology [CD-Rom].* Jenkintown, Pennsylvania: ©National Comprehensive Cancer Network, May 2005. To view the most recent and complete version of the guidelines, go online to www.nccn.org.*

40. Smith FA, Querques J, Levenson JL & Stern TA (2005). Psychiatric assessment and consultation. In JL Levenson (Ed.), *The American Psychiatric Publishing Textbook of Psychosomatic Medicine* (pp.3-36). Washington, DC: American Psychiatric Publishing, Inc.

41. Folstein MF, Folstein SE & McHugh PR (1975). "Mini-mental state". A practical method for grading the cognitive state of patients for the clinician. *Journal of Psychiatric Research, 12,* 189-198.

42. Bruera E & Neumann CM (1998). The uses of psychotropics in symptom management in advanced cancer. *Psycho-Oncology, 7,* 346-358.

43. Meyers CA, Weitzner MA, Valentine AD & Levin VA (1998). Methylphenidate therapy improves cognition, mood, and function of brain tumor patients. *Journal of Clinical Oncology, 16,* 2522-2527.

Substance Abuse

44. Colliver JD & Kopstein AN (1991). Trends in cocaine abuse reflected in emergency room episodes reported to DAWN. Drug Abuse Warning Network. *Public Health Reports, 106,* 59 68.

45. Gfroerer J & Brodsky M (1992). The incidence of illicit drug use in the United States, 1962 1989. *British Journal of Addiction, 87,* 1345.

46. Regier DA, Farmer ME, Rae DS, Locke BZ, Keith SJ, Judd LL, et al. (1990). Comorbidity of mental disorders with alcohol and other drug abuse. *Journal of the American Medical Association, 264,* 2511-2518.

47. Bruera E, Moyano J, Seifert L, Fainsinger RL, Hanson J & Suarez-Almazor M (1995). The frequency of alcoholism among patients with pain due to terminal cancer. *Journal of Pain and Symptom Management, 10,* 599.

48. Rinaldi RC, Steindler EM, Wilford BB & Goodwin D (1988). Clarification and standardization of substance abuse terminology. *Journal of the American Medical Association, 259,* 555.

49. Passik SD & Weinreb HJ (2000). Managing chronic nonmalignant pain: Overcoming obstacles to the use of opioids. *Advances in Therapy, 17,* 70-80.

50. Substance Abuse (DIS-15, and -16). Reproduced with permission from the *NCCN 1.2005 Distress Management, The Complete Library of NCCN Clinical Practice Guidelines in Oncology [CD-Rom].* Jenkintown, Pennsylvania: ©National Comprehensive Cancer Network, May 2005. To view the most recent and complete version of the guidelines, go online to www.nccn.org.*

51. Handelsman L, Stein JA, Bernstein DP, Oppenheim SE, Rosenblum A & Magura S (2000). A latent variable analysis of coexisting emotional deficits in substance abusers: Alexithymia, hostility, and PTSD. *Addictive Behaviors, 25,* 423-428.

Personality Disorders

52. American Psychiatric Association. (1994). *Diagnostic and statistical manual of mental disorders* (4th ed.). Washington, DC: Author.

53. Hay JL & Passik SD (2000). The cancer patient with borderline personality disorder: Suggestions for symptom-focused management in the medical setting. *Psycho-Oncology, 9*, 91-100.

54. Eysenck HJ (1987). The definition of personality disorders and the criteria appropriate for their descriptions. *Journal of Personality Disorders, 1*, 211-219.

55. Pinkofsky HB (1997). Mnemonics for DSM-IV personality disorders. *Psychiatric Services, 48*, 1197-1198.

56. Fishbain DA (1999). Approaches to treatment decisions for psychiatric comorbidity in the management of the chronic pain patient. *Medical Clinics of North America, 83*, 737-760.

57. Melartin TK, Rytsala HJ, Leskela US, Lestela-Mielonen PS, Sokero TP & Isometsa ET (2002). Current comorbidity of psychiatric disorders among DSM-IV major depressive disorder patients in psychiatric care in the Vantaa Depression Study. *Journal of Clinical Psychiatry, 63*, 126-34.

58. Hewitt M & Rowland JH (2002). Mental health service use among adult cancer survivors: Analyses of the national health interview survey. *Journal of Clinical Oncology, 20*, 4581-4590.

59. Personality Disorder (DIS-17). Reproduced with permission from the *NCCN 1.2005 Distress Management, The Complete Library of NCCN Clinical Practice Guidelines in Oncology [CD-Rom]*. Jenkintown, Pennsylvania: ©National Comprehensive Cancer Network, May 2005. To view the most recent and complete version of the guidelines, go online to www.nccn.org.*

7 Physical Symptom Management

Fatigue

Introduction

Definition: A common persistent, subjective sense of tiredness related to cancer or cancer treatment that interferes with usual functioning.[1]

Prevalence: 60-90% of individuals with cancer experience fatigue.[2,3] Fatigue persists after treatment, sometimes for years, in many cancer survivors.

Impact: Fatigue is the symptom that cancer patients report most frequently, describe as the most distressing, and which is associated with the most debilitating impact on functioning.[3]

Table 7.1   Fatigue Screening and Evaluation

One-Item Scale
NCCN recommended:
one-item, 0-10 screen
for fatigue[1]
	• Asks: "Since your last visit, how would you rate your fatigue on a scale of 0-10, with '0' being 'no fatigue' and '10' being 'most severe fatigue?'"
	• Scores can be grouped categorically according to fatigue severity:
	    0 = no fatigue
	    1 - 3 = mild fatigue
	    4 - 6 = moderate fatigue
	    7 - 10 = severe fatigue
	• Patients with scores of 4 or above should receive further evaluation.[4]

Validated Instruments	• Brief Fatigue Inventory (BFI)[5] • Fatigue Symptom Inventory (FSI)[6] • Functional Assessment of Chronic Illness Therapy- Fatigue Scale (FACIT-F)[7]

Table 7.2   Fatigue History

Onset	• "When did you first notice feeling fatigue?"
Current State	• "How would you rate your fatigue right now on a scale of 0 to 10?" • "How is your fatigue now compared to other times in your treatment?"
Level of Functioning	• "Describe a typical day for you." • "How much of the day do you spend in bed or resting?" • "Do you need to take naps?" • "Are you able to walk a block? ...climb stairs? ...drive? ...do housework?" • "Are you able to work? How many hours?"
Relation to Cancer Treatments	• "Did you notice any change in your fatigue—better or worse—during the treatment? How about in the few weeks right after the treatment?"
Exacerbating and Alleviating Factors	• "When was your fatigue the worst? What was going on around that time?" • "Does anything seem to make your fatigue worse? ...better?" • "Are naps helpful?"
Response to Past Interventions	• "What have you tried so far for your fatigue?" • "Has anyone recommend any treatments for your fatigue?" • "How did it work?" • "Did you have any side effects?"
Impact on Relationships and Social Support	• "Has your fatigue been stressful or frustrating for your relationships?" • "Has your fatigue made you want to spend more time by yourself?"

Table 7.3   Distinguishing Fatigue from Depression[8]

Fatigue	• Patients usually are able to derive some pleasure from activities that they normally find enjoyable. • Late afternoon as the most difficult time[9]
Depression	• Patients are unable to experience pleasure from experiences they usually enjoy.[10] • Morning is the most difficult time of the day. • Patients have suicidal thoughts and hopelessness. • Past history of major depression and/or family history of major depression may increase the likelihood of developing an episode of depression. • In cases of uncertainty, an empiric trial of antidepressant therapy may be best in order not to let a possible case of depression go untreated.

Table 7.4   Causes of Cancer-related Fatigue

Area	Assessment	Consults	Treatments
Anemia	Hemoglobin level		• For chemotherapy- related anemia, epoetin (Procrit) is recommended for hemoglobin levels less than 10 g/dl. If patient has hemoglobin level of 10-12 g/dl, consider using epoetin if symptomatic from fatigue. (ASCO Clinical Practice guidelines, www.asco.org)
Sleep Disturbance	Insomnia	Consider psychiatry consult for refractory insomnia	• Hypnotics such as *zolpidem* (Ambien®) • Short-acting benzodiazepines such as *oxazepam* (Serax®) • *Gabapentin* (Neurontin®)
	Inability to stay asleep		• Long-acting benzodiazepines such as clonazepam (Klonopin®) • *Mirtazapine* (Remeron®) • Sedating atypical antipsychotics such as *quetiapine* (Seroquel®), especially if on glucocorticoids
	Physical symptoms interfering with sleep		• Pain control • Trial of SSRI for hot flashes • Oxygen for SOB • Reduction of fluid intake during evening hours to limit bathroom trips
	Early morning awakenings	Mental health evaluation to rule out depression	• Consider antidepressant medications. (Cf. Chapter 4.)
	Snoring and daytime somnolence	Sleep study to rule out sleep apnea	• CPAP

(continued, next page)

Table 7.4   Causes of Cancer-related Fatigue (continued)

Emotional Distress	Distress Thermometer: "What is your distress level on a scale of 0-10?"	Scores of 4 or above on Distress Thermometer warrant evaluation for anxiety and depression	• Psychosocial support • Individual or group therapy • Medications for anxiety (cf. Chapter 4) and depression (cf. Chapter 6, Mood Disorders).
Pain	0-10 pain scale; Comprehensive pain assessment (see section on Pain in this chapter)	Pain Service; anaesthesia or neurosurgery for procedures	• Maximize pain control. (Cf. section on Pain in this chapter.)
Activity Level	History of exercise, functional abilities, and how patient spends a typical day	Physical Therapy	• Encourage increased physical activity and gentle exercise.
Nutrition	Weight; albumin level; eating history	Nutritionist	• Anti-emetics for nausea and vomiting • Trials of appetite stimulants such as *megestrol* (Megace®), *methylphenidate* (Ritalin®), *mirtazapine* (Remeron®) • Consideration of g-tube or parenteral nutrition
Medical Co-Morbidity (e.g. hypothyroidism, hypercalcemia, infection, cardiac disease, hepatic failure, renal disease)	Medical history; physical examination; laboratory and imaging studies	Internal medicine or appropriate specialists	• Treat any underlying co-morbid medical conditions. • Minimize sedating medications or switch to less sedating alternatives if possible.

Table 7.5   Fatigue Treatments

Specifics	*Precautions*
Medications	
methylphenidate (Ritalin®): Starting dose usually is 5 mg bid. Therapeutic range is 5 to 30 mg bid. (Daily extended release forms are available.)	• Common side effects include constipation, anorexia, headaches, nervousness, and difficulty sleeping. • May also elevate heart rate and blood pressure • May not be appropriate for patients with schizophrenia, bipolar disorder, delirium, and severe anxiety
dextroamphetamine (Dexedrine®): Starting dose usually is 5 mg bid. Therapeutic range is 5 to 30 mg bid.	• Common side effects include constipation, anorexia, headaches, nervousness, and difficulty sleeping. • May also elevate heart rate and blood pressure • May not be appropriate for patients with schizophrenia, bipolar disorder, delirium, and severe anxiety
modafinil (Provigil®): Starting dose usually is 100 to 200 mg/day. Therapeutic range is 100 to 400 mg/day.	• Common side effects include headache, insomnia, anxiety/nervousness, diarrhea, and dyspepsia.
Patient Education • Validate of fatigue as a common medical problem. • Place fatigue in context of patient's illness. (What are some of the causes?) • Explore patient's beliefs and worries about the fatigue. • Develop a plan together for monitoring and treating fatigue.	• Patients may be afraid to discuss fatigue with their care providers because of fears of being seen as too weak to receive treatment. They may fear that potentially life-saving treatment will be withheld.
Exercise • Exercise is the most evidence-based intervention. • Patients may need motivational interviewing to increase their physical activity.	• Patients may need to ratchet down their expectations as compared to before cancer. • Physical therapy may be helpful in developing a safe exercise program, especially in patients with physical limitations.

(continued, next page)

Table 7.5   Fatigue Treatments (continued)

Specifics	*Precautions*
Behavioral Management • Prioritizing activities • Problem solving around difficult tasks • Utilizing energy-saving strategies: monitoring variations in energy levels over the course of the day; trying to take advantage of patterns of higher energy	• Goal: Increase functionality with greater organization of activity without decreasing overall physical activity. • Decreasing overall physical activity could lead to further deconditioning.

Pain

Introduction

Pain is perhaps the symptom most feared by people with cancer and many patients may equate cancer with a painful death. Some patients, who may not even be experiencing pain, may express a desire to end their lives in the future when the pain becomes "too much."

Pain interferes with sleep, appetite, mood; and contributes to anxiety, fatigue, and poor quality of life. Barriers to pain management include fears of addiction. Pain is the fifth vital sign and should be assessed at each clinical encounter.

This chapter uses the NCCN Guidelines on Pain as a framework for a comprehensive approach to pain in the cancer patient.[II]

Table 7.6   Pain Screening and Evaluation

One-Item, 0-10 Scale	• "How much pain are you having, on a scale of 0 (no pain) to 10 (worst pain you can imagine)?"
	0 = no pain 4 - 6 = moderate pain
	1 - 3 = mild pain 7 - 10 = severe pain
	For a pain score of 5 or greater, re-evaluate or refer to a pain specialist.

(continued, next page)

Table 7.6   Pain Screening and Evaluation (continued)

Pain Assessment Tools	• Over 100 validated instruments are available. • Brief Pain Inventory by Cleeland (eight-item questionnaire that assesses the presence, location, and severity of pain; interference caused by pain; and response pain treatment)[12] • McGill Pain Questionnaire by Melzack (twenty-item questionnaire that assesses sensory, affective, and qualitative aspects of pain)[13]

Comprehensive Pain Assessment[11]	• **Pain intensity:** How severe is the pain on the scale of 0 - 10?
	• **Location** of the pain
	• **Quality** of the pain: Ask the patient to describe what the pain feels like.
	  • Aching, stabbing, throbbing, pressure suggests somatic pain.
	  • Gnawing, cramping, aching, or sharp may suggest visceral pain, depending on the location.
	  • Sharp, tingling, burning, or shooting suggests neuropathic pain.
	• **Pain history**
	  • When did it start?
	  • How long has it been present?
	  • Has it changed in any ways?
	  • Is it intermittent or constant?
	  • Do you have other symptoms?
	  • What makes the pain worse? ...better?
	  • What has been tried to treat the pain? Has it helped? Are there side effects? What are the scheduled doses?
	• **Etiology:** Underlying causes of the pain must be identified and treated when possible. Emergency problems like spinal cord compression or infection must be treated immediately.
	• **Medical history:** Pain should be evaluated in the context of the cancer and other significant medical illnesses, as well as current medications including over-the-counter and complementary substances.
	• **Psychosocial issues:** Evaluate level of distress, psychiatric disorders, history of substance abuse, and level of support from others.
	  • ***Support:*** Who does the patient have for support? Family and others available? Is anyone helping to manage the pain and medications at home? Reliable?
	  • ***Distress:*** How much distress is the pain causing? Is the pain bearable or unbearable? Does the diffuseness of the distress suggest emotional suffering rather than nociception? What does the patient think that the pain means (e.g. tumor spread)? What are cultural, spiritual or religious concerns about pain?

(continued, next page)

Table 7.6   Pain Screening and Evaluation (continued)

Comprehensive Pain Assessment (continued)[11]	• **Psychosocial issues (continued)**
	  • *Psychiatric illness:*
	    Anxiety - Conditioned anticipatory anxiety may begin before dressing changes or painful walking. Patients may seek analgesics to allay anxiety or to treat insomnia rather than pain. Panic attacks may cause pain in chest or stomach.
	    Depression - When patients have clinical depression, all pain is worse. Patients in pain are more likely to have secondary depression. Assess history of depression and current depressive symptoms (sleep disturbance; loss of interest; guilt/hopelessness/helplessness; low energy; concentration difficulties; appetite changes; psychomotor retardation; suicidal ideation).
	    Chronic Pain Syndromes - Includes fibromyalgia, pelvic pain syndrome, suggesting predisposing patterns of pain behavior.
	    Substance Abuse - Patients with psychiatric or opiate abuse histories may require higher doses due to tolerance. Addictive behavior: Use caution in patients with a history of drug dependence or alcoholism. (Cf. Chapter 6, Substance Abuse.)
	• **Physical examination** with laboratory and imaging studies

Risk Factors for Under-Treatment	• Children; elderly; women; minorities (language, cultural barriers) • History of substance abuse; psychiatric illness; neuropathic pain

Table 7.7   Pain Treatment[11]

Initial Treatment	• Screening for pain at each visit with the one-item and 0 - 10 scale. • If the pain score is greater than 0, evaluate with the comprehensive pain assessment; if above 5, pain must be re-evaluated or referred. • Treat underlying causes of the pain while providing analgesia. • Initiate pain medications based on the intensity of the pain. • *Severe pain* (score 7-10): Rapidly titrate short-acting opioids. (Cf. Table 7.9.) For patients not on opioids, administer 5-10 mg of oral immediate-release morphine sulfate and reassess after 60 minutes. If pain is unchanged, double the dose and repeat until pain score decreases by at least 50%. If pain score decreases by less than 50%, repeat the same dose and reassess. After pain score is decreased by at least 50%, calculate the total amount given over 4 hours for the "effective 4 hour dose." If the patient is already on opioids, continue long-acting opioids and increase the dose of daily oral morphine equivalent by 30-40%. Reassess after 60 minutes and titrate the dose as described above. Intravenous opioids can be titrated starting at 2-5 mg IV. Reassess after fifteen minutes. (continued, next page)

Table 7.7   Pain Treatment (continued)[11]

Initial Treatment (continued)	• *Moderate pain* (score 4 - 6): If the patient is not on opioids, administer 5 - 10 mg of oral immediate-release morphine sulfate or equivalent and reassess in 4 hours. If the pain score has decreased by less than 50%, increase the dose by 25 - 50% and repeat assessment in 4 hours. If the pain score decreased by at least 50%, this is the "effective 4 hour dose." If the patient is already on opioids, increase the dose of daily oral morphine equivalent by 25 - 50%. Reassess in 4 hours and titrate the dose based on response as described above.
	• *Mild pain* (score 1 - 3): Consider NSAID or acetaminophen without opioid if patient is not on analgesics (cf. Table 7.10). Consider titrating short-acting opioids according to algorithm for moderate pain.
	• Utilize strategies for managing side effects from the medications such as prophylactic bowel regimens and antiemetics for narcotics.
	• Monitor and adjust medications for sedation and delirium (cf. Chapter 6, Delirium). Follow the patient's sleep pattern and ability to think clearly. Delirium interferes with orientation, concentration, memory, level of consciousness. Opioids at higher doses increase the risk of delirium. Concomitant benzodiazepines raise the risk of delirium.
	• To reduce the risk of delirium, increase narcotics slowly, e.g. 25 - 50%, then decrease as tolerated to diminish problems with cognition and delirium.
	• Older patients are more sensitive to these side effects.
	• The narcotic may accumulate, depending upon its half-life. Doses should be reduced gradually if cause of pain has been treated or if the patient has adequate pain relief.
	• Use psychotropic medications to augment narcotics, e.g. neuroleptics for anxiety or cognitive impairment such as *haloperidol* (Haldol®) or *quetiapine* (Seroquel®); stimulants for alertness such as *methylphenidate* (Ritalin®), *dextroamphetamine* (Dexedrine®), and *modafinil* (Provigil®).
	• Provide education and psychosocial support.
Conversion to Longer Acting Opioids	• Once pain is stable on immediate-release opioids, consider switching to longer-acting opioids.
	• Calculate dose based on 24-hour requirement and prescribe equivalent dose of extended-release *morphine sulfate* (MS Contin®), extended release *oxycodone hydrochloride* (OxyContin®), or *transdermal fentanyl* (Duragesic®).
	• Provide rescue doses of short-acting opioids for breakthrough pain. Use immediate release forms of the long-acting opioid whenever possible and allow rescue doses of 10 - 20% of the total 24-hour dosage q. one hour as needed. If using *transdermal fentanyl* (Duragesic®), the 24-hour oral morphine equivalent is twice the hourly dose of fentanyl in mcgs.

(continued, next page)

Table 7.7   Pain Treatment (continued)[11]

Worsening Pain on Stable Treatment	• Continue screening for pain with the one-item and 0 - 10 scale.
	• If pain appears to be worsening, evaluate with comprehensive pain assessment.
	• Treat underlying causes of pain while providing analgesia.
	• If the patient is taking opioids, increase both around the clock and as needed doses based on the intensity of the pain.
	   • Severe pain (score 7 - 10): Consider increasing dose by 50-100%.
	   • Moderate pain (score 4 - 6): Consider increasing dose by 25-50%.
	   • Mild pain (score 1 - 3): Consider increasing dose by 25%.
	• If the patient is not on opioids, consider starting opioids and titrating dose according to intensity of pain.

Special Pain Issues	• **Bone pain**: In addition to trials of NSAIDS or opioids, other interventions are available for bone pain. If the pain is diffuse, bisphosphonates, hormonal or chemotherapy for responsive tumors, glucocorticoids, and/or systemic administration of radioisotopes is beneficial. If the pain is localized, consider local radiation therapy or nerve block. For resistant pain, consider referral to anesthesia, orthopedic or neurosurgery. • **Neuropathic pain**: Narcotics and other classes of medications, particularly antidepressants, show some efficacy (cf. Table 7.11) .[14] Smaller doses of antidepressants may be effective, but many times these medications may need to be titrated to doses similar to the treatment of depression. • **Pain from inflammation:** Pain from inflammation may be best treated by decreasing the inflammation with NSAIDS or glucocorticoids. • **Nerve compression or inflammation**: A trial of glucocorticoids is indicated.

Table 7.8   Consultations for Pain

Procedures	• If pain is not adequately controlled by analgesics or if the side effects have become intolerable, a referral to anesthesia or neurosurgery for a pain relieving procedure may be indicated. • Consultation may also be sought early in treatment if the pain is localized to an area that would be relieved by a nerve block. • Common procedures are regional infusions to epidural, intrathecal, or regional plexus; neurodestructive procedures for well-localized pain syndromes; and percutaneous vertebroplasty.

(continued, next page)

Table 7.8   Consultations for Pain (continued)

Non-pharmacological Consultations	• *Physical modalities* are heat or ice; ultrasonic stimulation; transcutaneous electrical nerve stimulation (TENS); acupuncture, and massage. A physical therapy consultation might be useful for better positioning; strengthening compensatory muscle groups; and supplying bed, bath, and walking supports. • *Cognitive treatments* are relaxation training; distraction; hypnosis; and cognitive behavioral therapy (cf. Table 7.12).[15] (Cf. Chapter 5.) • *Emotional support and education* for the patient and family is essential. A sustained, positive relationship to the treating physician is the cornerstone of management. • A referral to a psychiatrist, psychologist, or social worker may be particularly helpful in evaluating and treating mood and anxiety symptoms related to the pain, delirium, sedation, and other mental status changes. Cognitive behavioral therapy is best delivered by a trained therapist. This approach is helpful in chronic pain not fully responsive to medications.

Table 7.9   Opioid Medications - Adapted from NCCN Guidelines[11]

Opioid*	Oral Dose	IV Dose	Dose Frequency	Half Life
codeine	100 mg	50 mg	q 3 - 4 hr	2.9 hr
hydrocodone (Vicodin®)	15 mg	n/a	q 3 - 4 hr	3.5 - 4.1 hr
oxycodone (OxyFast®)	7.5 - 10 mg	n/a	q 3 - 4 hr	3.2 hr
morphine	15 mg	5 mg	q 3 - 4 hr	1.5 - 2 hr
hydromorphone (Dilaudid®)	4 mg	0.75 - 1.5 mg	q 3 - 4 hr	2.5 hr
levorphanol (Levo-Dromorane®)	2 mg	1 mg	q 6 - 8 hr	11 - 30 hr
methadone (Dolophine®)	10 mg	5 mg	q 6 - 8 hr	15 - 30 hr
fentanyl (Duragesic®)	n/a	50 mcg	q 2 - 3 hr, transdermal q 48 - 72 hr	1.5 - 6 hr

* Side effects include constipation, nausea, and vomiting, drowsiness, sedation, confusion, respiratory depression and hypotension.

Table 7.10 Anti-Inflammatory and Non-Narcotic Medications - Adapted from NCCN Guidelines[11]

Medication	Usual Dose	Side Effects
ibuprofen (Motrin®)	400 mg qid (maximum daily dose = 3,200 mg)	Epigastric pain; gastric or duodenal ulcers; GI bleeding; tinnitus; nausea and vomiting; nervousness; rash
Choline and magnesium salicylate combinations	1.5 - 4.5 g in 3 divided doses	Gastritis; GI bleeding; nausea; tinnitus
salsalate (Salflex®)	2 - 3 g in 2 - 3 divided doses	Nausea; GI bleeding; tinnitus; hearing impairment; hepatic dysfunction; decreased creatinine clearance
acetaminophen (Tylenol®)	650 mg q4 hr (maximum daily dose = 4 g)	Hepatic dysfunction; hepatic failure; renal disease; nephropathy; anemia; SIADH; transient hypothermia

Table 7.11 Medications for Neuropathic Pain* [14]

Class	Medication	Starting Dose	Usual Dose	Side Effects
Tricyclic antidepressants	amitriptyline (Elavil®)	10 - 25 mg qhs	10 - 200 mg qhs	Constipation; dry mouth; blurred vision; sedation; urinary retention; orthostatic hypotension; tachycardia; cardiac conduction changes; leukopenia; thrombocytopenia
	desipramine (Norpramin®)	10 - 25 mg qhs	100 - 300 mg qhs	
	doxepin (Sinequan®)	10 - 25 mg qhs	10 - 150 mg qhs	
	nortriptyline (Pamelor®)	10 - 25 mg qhs	10 - 100 mg qhs	
Serotonin and norepinephrine reuptake inhibitors: antidepressants	venlafaxine (Effexor®)	37.5 - 75 mg/day	75 - 300 mg/day	Constipation; nausea and vomiting; anorexia; somnolence; sweating; sedation; sexual dysfunction; hyper-tension w/ venlafaxine
	duloxetine (Cymbalta®)	20 mg/day	20 - 60 mg/day	

* Cf. Table 7.7.

(continued, next page)

Table 7.11 Medications for Neuropathic Pain (continued)

Class	Medication	Starting Dose	Usual Dose	Side Effects
Atypical antidepressant	buproprion (Wellbutrin®)	100 mg bid	200 - 450 mg/day (divide dose of immediate release to no more than 150 mg at one time)	Agitation; tremor; sweating; headache; constipation; dry mouth; blurred vision; nausea; increased risk for seizures; slow-release SR (12 h half-life) and XL (24 hour half-life)
Anti-convulsants	carbamazepine (Tegretol®)	50 - 100 mg bid	50 - 1200 mg/day	Nausea and vomiting; sedation; blurred vision; nystagmus; rash; blood pressur changes; renal toxicity; SIADH; bone marrow dysfunction; leukopenia; leukocytosis; thrombocytopenia
	gabapentin (Neurontin®)	100 - 300 mg tid	300 - 3600 mg/day	Sedation; ataxia; blurred vision; peripheral edema
	lamotrogine (Lamictal®)	25 mg qhs (increase daily dose by 25 mg every 2 weeks and no faster)	50 - 200 mg/day	Ataxia; sedation; blurred vision; headache; nausea; rash; Stevens-Johnson Syndrome. Rash related to rate of increase.
Opioid analgesic	tramadol (Ultram®)	25 mg qd (increase daily dose by 25 mg every 3 days)	50 - 100 mg q 6 hours (maximum dose 400 mg/day)	Constipation; diarrhea; nausea and vomiting; dizziness; sedation; confusion; headache; pruritis
Local anesthetic	lidocaine patch (5%) (Xylocaine®)		Up to 3 patches at once, no more than 12 hours in a 24 hour period	Localized erhythema; CNS excitation; confusion; depression; dizziness; bradycardia; hypotension

Table 7.12 Cognitive Interventions for Pain Management*

Relaxation Training	Relaxation techniques: imagery (described below) or progressive muscle relaxation. In progressive muscle relaxation, the patient actively tenses and then relaxes specific muscle groups. Usually starts with feet, progressing systematically to the muscles of the head.
Imagery	Relaxation with concentration on a pleasant mental image, such as the patient's favorite place. Imagery may be more successful if all senses are involved in imagining the scene.
Distraction	Focusing attention away from pain and onto another thought or activity such as listening to music.
Hypnosis	Deep relaxation followed by imagery and suggestions such as transforming the pain into another sensation like warmth.
Biofeedback	Using physiological monitors, such as heart rate and blood pressure monitors and electromyogram (EMG), to train patients to better control their pain through relaxation.
Cognitive-behavioral Therapy	Re-framing thoughts about pain and distress; problem solving the difficulties caused by pain; finding alternative coping strategies that are more adaptive; and treatment of anxiety and depressive symptoms that may be contributing to pain.

* Cf. Chapter 5.

Nausea and Vomiting

Introduction

Most patients with cancer fear chemotherapy because of possible nausea and vomiting. Although anti-emetic therapies have greatly improved chemotherapy-related nausea and vomiting, they remain common symptoms affecting up to 70-80% of patients receiving chemotherapy.[16] Sometimes nausea and vomiting are so severe that patients dread their treatments or decide to discontinue. Conditioned nausea and vomiting may recur as anticipatory symptoms; they can persist for years with reminders of the treatment. Nausea and vomiting not only interfere with a patient's quality of life, they also can cause medical complications such as metabolic imbalances, poor nutrition, aspiration pneumonia, esophageal tears, and surgical wound dehiscence.[17]

This chapter utilizes the NCCN Guidelines for Antiemesis as a framework for approaching the clinical problem of nausea and vomiting.[18] Three broad categories of nausea are: chemotherapy-induced, radiation-induced, and non-treatment-related nausea.

Table 7.13 Chemotherapy-Induced Nausea

Type of Nausea	Risk factors	Treatments
Acute Onset Develops within minutes to hours after receiving chemotherapy, peaks in 5-6 hours and usually resolves within 24 hours	• Emetogenic potential of chemotherapy agent, type and likelihood (see Table 7.16) • Previous episodes of nausea and vomiting with chemotherapy • Younger age • Female • History of motion sickness • Expectation that chemotherapy will cause nausea • Less likely with history of alcoholism chemotherapy will cause nausea	• Prophylactic treatment with anti-emetics
Delayed Emesis Develops 24 hours after chemotherapy administration, may peak in 48-72 hours and last 6-7 days	• More likely with cisplatin, carboplatin, cyclophosphamide, and doxorubicin • Younger age • Female	• Prophylactic treatment with combination of metoclopramide (Reglan®), steroids, and a 5-HT3 antagonist • Possible addition of NK1 antagonist. Continuation of antiemetics for 7 days after chemotherapy[17]
Anticipatory Nausea (experienced by 14 - 40% of patients) Occurs before the administration of chemotherapy in patients who previously had chemotherapy and emesis	• Negative experience of nausea and vomiting after prior chemotherapy treatment; younger age; possible association with history of anxiety or depression; sweating, generalized weakness, or feeling warm all over after last chemotherapy session[19]	• Pretreatment with lorazepam (Ativan®) • behavioral management: relaxation, distraction, hypnosis, systematic desensitization

Table 7.14 Risks of Emesis for Specific Chemotherapy Agents - Adapted from NCCN Guidelines[18]

High Risk, Level 5 (> 90% frequency of emesis)

Carmustine > 250 mg/m^2	Dacarbazine
Cisplatin > 50 mg/m^2	Mechlorethamine
Cyclophosphamide > 1,500 mg/m^2	Streptozocin

Moderate Risk, Level 4 (60 - 90% frequency of emesis)

Amifostine > 500 mg/m^2	Dactinomycin
Busulfan > 4 mg/d	Doxorubicin > 60 mg/m^2
Carboplatin	Epirubicin > 90 mg/m^2
Carmustine < 250 mg/m^2	Melphalan > 50 mg/m^2
Cisplatin < 50 mg/m^2	Methotrexate > 1,000 mg/m^2
Cyclophosphamide > 750 mg/m^2 and < 1,500 mg/m^2	Procarbazine (oral)
Cytarabine > 1 mg/m^2	

Moderate Risk, Level 3 (30 - 60% frequency of emesis)

Amifostine > 300 to < 500 mg/m^2	Ifosfamide
Arsenic trioxide	Interleukin-2 (IL-2) > 12 - 15 million units/m^2
Cyclophosphamide < 750 mg/m^2	Irinotecan
Cyclophosphamide (oral)	Lomustine
Doxorubicin 20 to < 60 mg/m^2	Methotrexate 250 - 1,000 mg/m^2
Epirubicin < 90 mg/m^2	Mitoxanthrone < 15 mg/m^2
Hexamethylmelamine (oral)	Oxaliplatin > 75 mg/m^2
Idarubicin	

Low Risk, Level 2 (10 - 30% frequency of emesis)

Amifostine < 300 mg/m^2	Doxorubicin (liposomal)	Mitomycin
Bexarotene	Etoposide	Paclitaxel
Cytarabine 100 - 200 mg/m^2	Fluorouricil (5-FU) < 1,000 mg/m^2	Temozolomide
Capecitabine	Gemcitabine	Topotecan
Docetaxel	Methotrexate > 50 mg/m^2 < 250 mg/m^2	

Minimal Risk, Level 1 (< 10% frequency of emesis)

Alemtuzumab	Fludarabine	Rituximab
Asparaginase	Gefitinib	Thioguanine (oral)
Interferon-alpha	Gemtuzumab ozogamicin	Trastuzumab
Bleomycin	Hydoxyurea	Valrubicin
Bortezomib	Imatinib mesylate	Vinblastine
Chlorambucil (oral)	Melphalan (oral low-dose)	Vincristine
Dexrazoxane	Methotrexate < 50 mg	Vinorelbine
Denileukin diftitox	Pentostatin	

Table 7.15 Radiation-induced Nausea and Vomiting

- Whole body, chest, head and neck regions or upper abdominal radiation therapy
- Higher daily fractional dose of radiotherapy, the total dose, and the amount of irradiated tissue increase the risk of developing radiation-induced nausea.

Table 7.16 Causes of Non-treatment-related Nausea and Vomiting

- Partial or complete bowel obstruction
- Vestibular dysfunction
- Brain metastases
- Electrolyte imbalance: hypercalcemia, hyperglycemia, hyponatremia
- Uremia
- Concomitant medications, e.g., opiates
- Gastroparesis, tumor or chemotherapy-induced
- Psychophysiologic: Usually is an anxiety disorder or major depression with somatic symptoms. If patients do not respond to usual treatment, consider a referral to a mental health clinician, especially if there are anxious or depressive symptoms. Although many antidepressants, particularly the selective serotonin reuptake inhibitors (SSRI's), may have nausea as a potential side effects, they may be the treatment of choice in these cases.

Treatments for Nausea and Vomiting

Table 7.17 Anti-emetic Medications

Class	Medications	Side Effects
5-HT3 antagonists	dolasetron (Anzemet®) granisetron (Kytril®) ondansetron (Zofran®) palonosetron (Aloxi®)	Constipation; abdominal pain; dizziness; fatigue; malaise; headache; blurred vision; elevated liver function tests
Corticosteroids	dexamethasone (Decadron®) methylprednisolone (Medrol®)	Mood changes (insomnia, euphoria, irritability, or depression); GI distress; hypertension; skin atrophy; increased risk for infection; osteoporosis; cataracts; Cushing's syndrome
Benzodiazepines	lorazepam (Ativan®)	Sedation; dizziness; confusion; unsteadiness
NK-1 antagonists	aprepitant (Emend®)	Sedation; fatigue; hiccups

(continued, next page)

Table 7.17 Anti-emetic Medications (continued)

Class	Medications	Side Effects
Cannabinoids	dronabinol (Marinol®)	Confusion; depersonalization; euphoria; paranoid reaction; impaired coordination; changes in blood pressure; palpitations; tachycardia; vasodialation/flushing
Phenothiazines	prochlorperazine (Compazine®)	Akathisia; dystonic reactions; Parkinsonism; tardive dyskinesia; blurred vision; ocular changes; constipation; suicidal ideation; orthostatic hypotension; QT prolongation; leukopenia; thrombocytopenia; neuroleptic malignant syndrome (rare)
Butyrophenones	haloperidol (Haldol®) droperidol (Inapsine®)	Akathisia; dystonic reactions; Parkinsonism; tardive dyskinesia; blurred vision; ocular changes; constipation; suicidal ideation; orthostatic hypotension; QT prolongation; leukopenia; thrombocytopenia; neuroleptic malignant syndrome (rare)
Substituted benzamides	metoclopramide (Reglan®)	Constipation; sedation; dystonic reaction; restlessness; fluid retention; tremors
Atypical antipsychotics	olanzapine (Zyprexa®)	Sedation; dizziness; orthostatic hypotension; akathisia; elevated liver function tests; weight gain; neuroleptic malignant syndrome (rare)

Table 7.18 Behavioral Management of Nausea and Vomiting[19]

Symptom monitoring	For refractory nausea	Patient charts episodes of nausea and vomiting with details of onset, duration, exacerbating and alleviating factors, relation to medications and oral intake. May help to give patient a sense of control over the symptom and make environmental modifications to lessen nausea.
Progressive muscle relaxation	For acute onset and delayed emesis; may be less effective for anticipatory nausea	Actively tensing and then relaxing specific muscle groups, usually starting with feet and progressing systematically to the muscles of the head; sometimes done with guided imagery

(continued, next page)

Table 7.18 Behavioral Management of Nausea and Vomiting (continued)[19]

Systematic Desensitization	For anticipatory nausea	Identification of situation that causes the most nausea; list of cues for development of nausea; order cues from least to most nausea causing; gradual exposure to cues in hierarchical order starting with the least nausea causing; development of alternative responses for nausea for each cue with the goal of mastering the full situation
Hypnosis	For anticipatory nausea	Deep relaxation followed by imagery and suggestions such as successfully completing the activities of chemotherapy without developing nausea or vomiting
Cognitive Distraction	For anticipatory nausea; also could be used for acute onset and delayed emesis	Focusing attention away from nausea and onto another thought or activity, such as video games or music

Sexual Dysfunction[20,21]

Sexuality is an integral part of human life with the potential to create new life and fosters intimacy and shared pleasure in a relationship. It is an important part of health and general well being that cancer and cancer treatment can alter significantly.[22,23,24] This demonstrates to the patient that the clinician is open to questions and concerns about sexuality. Using Annon's PLISSIT Model of sexual assessment,[23] the clinician can open the discussion about sexuality with the aid of open-ended questions.

Table 7.19 Annon's PLISSIT Model[25]

Permission	Give permission to talk and think about sexuality and cancer at the same time: "What changes have you noticed sexually?" "Sexually, how are things going?" "Tell me about any sexual changes." "How has this affected you sexually?"
Limited Information	Tell the patient about sexual side effects: Erectile dysfunction, alopecia, alibido, vaginal dryness, menopausal symptoms.

(continued, next page)

Table 7.19 Annon's PLISSIT Model (continued)[25]

Specific Suggestions	Make suggestions to help with sexual dysfunction i.e., vaginal lubricants and moisturizers; medications, position changes, sensate focusing, safer sex.
Intensive Therapy	Refer to marital therapist, sexual therapist or psychotherapist.

Table 7.20 Phases of Sexual Function and Causes of Dysfunction[26]

Phases - Description and *Dysfunction*	Causes of Dysfunction	
Libido - Instinctual; multi-determined process; urge for or interest in sexual intercourse; trigger for remaining sexual phases; controlled by testosterone *Disinterest in sexual activity; absence of sexual fantasies*	• Anxiety • Body image • Chemotherapy • Depression • Fatigue • Hormones	• Medications • Menopause • Pain • Prostate cancer[27] • Relationship changes
Arousal - Increase in heart rate, respiratory rate, blood pressure and pelvic blood volume; in women, vaginal lubrication and swelling of genital tissues; in men, penile erection. *In women, vaginal dryness; in men, erectile dysfunction (consistent inability to obtain and/or maintain an erection sufficient for satisfactory sexual relation)*	• Anxiety • Body image • Chemotherapy • Depression • Dyspareunia • Fatigue • Medications • Menopause	• Neuropathies • Pain • Surgery for gynecological, prostate or rectal/anal cancers • Radiation to pelvic area
Orgasm - Rhythmic contraction of smooth muscles in and around the genitals; sense of physical pleasure and release; in men, ejaculation *Delayed; absent; happens too fast; retrograde or dry ejaculation*	• Anxiety • Chemotherapy • Depression • Fatigue • Medications	• Menopause • Pain • Radiation to pelvic area • Surgery to pelvic organs
Resolution - Period after orgasm; muscles relax, blood leaves genitals; penis flaccid, vaginal lubrication ends **Refractory period -** Length of time for the penis to "reset" and another erection to be possible *Refractory period lasting a day or more*	• Anxiety • Depression • Medications • Surgery	

Table 7.21 Factors Affecting Sexual Function[28]

Physical Changes
- Alopecia
- Anemia
- Central nervous system changes[29]
- Fatigue
- Hormone imbalances
- Immunosuppression
- Insomnia
- Pain
- Menopausal symptoms
- Muscle atrophy
- Shortness of breath
- Sterility
- Thrombocytopenia

Nutritional disturbances affecting ability for and interest in kissing and being touched[30]
- Anorexia
- Constipation
- Diarrhea
- Dry mouth
- Mucositis
- Nausea
- Vomiting
- Taste alterations associated with treatment

Psychological factors
- Adopting the 'patient' role (asexual)
- Altered body image
- Feelings of anxiety, depression, and anger
- Fears of death, rejection by partner, loss of control
- Guilt regarding behavior imagined as the cause of a disease or disability
- Reassignment of priorities[31]

Social and interpersonal factors
- Communication difficulties regarding feelings or sexuality
- Difficulty initiating sexual activity after a period of abstinence
- Fear of physically damaging an ill or disabled partner
- Lack of a partner
- Lack of privacy[31]

Table 7.22 Treatment of Sexual Dysfunction

Alibido (hypoactive sexual desire)
- Medicate physical symptoms (pain, nausea, etc.)
- Treat anxiety and depression or change antidepressants, e.g. *buproprion* (Wellbutrin®)
- Refer to sexual therapist
- Regular exercise
- Schedule sexual encounters
- Testosterone supplement or refer to endocrinologist
- Estrogen supplements (Estring® or vaginal estrogen cream)
- L-arginine for women who can't take estrogen

(continued, next page)

Table 7.22 Treatment of Sexual Dysfunction (continued)

Female sexual arousal disorder
- Vaginal lubricants and moisturizers
- EROS-CTD®- a vacuum device for females
- Sensate focus exercises
- Vibrators
- Vaginal dilators
- Positional change
- Treatment for depression and anxiety

Male erectile disorder
- Oral medications, e.g. *sildenafil* (Viagra®), *vardenafil* (Lavitra®), *tadalafil* (Cialis®)
- Transuretheral suppository, e.g. *alprostadil* (MUSE®)
- Vacuum constriction device
- Penile implant
- Penile injections
- Penile band
- Vibrators
- Positional change

Orgasmic disorder
- Change antidepressants (SSRIs can delay orgasm; consider substituting *burpropion* (Wellbutrin®)
- Vibrators
- Sensate focusing
- Self stimulation
- Positional change
- Refer to sexual therapist.
- Psychostimulants, e.g. *modafinil* (Provigil®), *methaphenadate* (Ritalin®)

Table 7.23 Referral Resources for Sexual Dysfunction

Referrals	Reason
Bowel management specialist	Diarrhea; constipation
Cardiologist	Assess cardiac function for *sildenafil* (Viagra®), *tadalafil* (Cialis®), *vardenafil* (Lavitra®)
Endocrinologist	Hormone, thyroid replacement; fertility issues
Fatigue specialist	Manage fatigue
Marital therapist[32]	Marital issues
Nutritionist	Weight control, loss; bowel problems; nausea
Pain specialist	Pain control
Psychiatrist	Depression; anxiety; adjustment disorder
Psychologist	Behavioral therapy
Sexual therapist	Sexual therapy, www.aasect.org, www.therapistlocator.net
Social worker	Housing; therapy

References

Fatigue

1. NCCN 2.2005 *Cancer-Related Fatigue, The Complete Library of NCCN Clinical Practice Guidelines in Oncology [CD-Rom].* Jenkintown, Pennsylvania: ©National Comprehensive Cancer Network, May 2005. To view the most recent and complete version of the guidelines, go online to www.nccn.org.*

2. Curt GA, Breitbart W, Cella, Groopman JE, Horning SJ, Johnson DH, et al. (2000). Impact of cancer-related fatigue on the lives of patients: New findings from the Fatigue Coalition. *Oncologist,* 5, 353-360.

3. Cella D, Davis K, Breitbart W, Curt G & Fatigue Coalition. (2001). Cancer-related fatigue: Prevalence of proposed diagnostic criteria in a United States sample of cancer survivors. *Journal of Clinical Oncology,* 19, 3385-3391.

4. Pirl WF, Temel J, Cashavelly B, and Lynch TJ. (2005). One-Item Scale is Valid for Rapid Screening of Fatigue in Thoracic Oncology Patients (abstract). *Proceedings of the American Society of Clinical Oncology Meeting* 2005: 748.

5. Mendoza TR, Wang XS, Cleeland CS, Morissey M, Johnson BA, Wendt JK, et al. (1999). The rapid assessment of fatigue severity in cancer patients: Use of the Brief Fatigue Inventory. *Cancer,* 85, 1186-1196.

6. Hann DM, Jacobsen PB, Azzarello LM, Martin SC, Curran SL, Fields KK, et al. (1998). Measurement of fatigue in cancer patients: Development and validation of the Fatigue Symptom Inventory. *Quality of Life Research,* 7, 301-310.

7. Cella D, Lai JS, Chang CH, Peterman A & Slavin M (2002). Fatigue in cancer patients compared with fatigue in the general population. *Cancer,* 94, 528-538.

8. Jacobsen PB, Donovan KA & Weitzner MA (2003). Distinguishing fatigue and depression in patients with cancer. *Seminars in Clinical Neuropsychiatry,* 8, 229-240.

9. Booth-Jones M, Donovan KA & Jacobsen PB (2004). Relationship of temporal variation in fatigue to depression in cancer patients [Abstract]. *Psycho-Oncology,* 13, S18.

10. Reuter K & Harter M (2003). Fatigue and/or depression? Examination of the construct validity of CRF. *Psycho-Oncology,* 12(Suppl.), 259-260.

Pain

11. NCCN 2.2005 *Adult Cancer Pain, The Complete Library of NCCN Clinical Practice Guidelines in Oncology [CD-Rom]*. Jenkintown, Pennsylvania: ©National Comprehensive Cancer Network, May 2005. To view the most recent and complete version of the guidelines, go online to www.nccn.org.*

12. Cleeland CS & Ryan KM (1994). Pain assessment: Global use of the Brief Pain Inventory. *ANNALS Academy of Medicine Singapore, 23*, 129-138.

13. Melzack R (1975). The McGill Pain Questionnaire: Major properties and scoring methods. *Pain, 1*, 277-299.

14. Dworkin RH, Backonja M, Rowbotham MC, Allen RR, Argoff CR, Bennett GJ, et al. (2003). Advances in neuropathic pain. *Archives of Neurology, 60*, 1524-1534.

15. Breitbart W & Payne DK (1998). Pain. In W Breitbart (Ed.), Management of specific symptoms. In JC Holland (Ed.), *Psycho-Oncology* (pp. 450-467). New York: Oxford University Press.

Nausea and Vomiting

16. Morran C, Smith DC, Anderson DA & McArdle CS (1979). Incidence of nausea and vomiting with cytotoxic chemotherapy: A prospective randomised trial of antiemetics. *British Medical Journal, 1*, 1323-1324.

17. Roffman JL & Pirl WF (2003). The use of antipsychotic medication in chemotherapy-induced nausea and vomiting. *Expert Review of Neurotherapeutics, 3*, 77-84.

18. NCCN 1.2005 Antiemesis, The Complete Library of NCCN Clinical Practice Guidelines in Oncology [CD-Rom]. Jenkintown, Pennsylvania: ©National Comprehensive Cancer Network, May 2005. To view the most recent and complete version of the guidelines, go online to www.nccn.org.*

19. Morrow GR, Roscoe JA & Hickok JT (1998). Nausea and vomiting. In W Breitbart (Ed.), Management of specific symptoms. In JC Holland (Ed.), *Psycho-Oncology* (pp. 476-484). New York: Oxford University Press.

Sexual Dysfunction

20. Laumann EO, Paik A, Rosen RC (1999) Sexual dysfunction in the United States: prevalence and predictors. [Published erratum JAMA 281(13):1174.] JAMA. 281(6):537-544.

21. Levine SB (1998). *Sexuality in mid-life*. New York: Plenum Press.Auchincloss SS (1991). Sexual dysfunction after cancer treatment. *Journal of Psychosocial Oncology, 9*, 23-41.

22. Auchincloss SS (1991). Sexual dysfunction after cancer treatment. *Journal of Psychosocial Oncology, 9*, 23-41.

23. Hughes MK (2000). Sexuality and the cancer survivor: A silent coexistence. *Cancer Nursing, 23*, 477-482.

24. Nusbaum MR, Gamble G, Skinner B & Heiman J (2000) The high prevalence of sexual concerns among women seeking routine gynecological care. *Journal of Family Practice, 49*, 229-32.

25. Annon JS (1976). The PLISSIT Model: A proposed conceptual scheme for the behavioral treatment of sexual problems. *Journal of Sex Education and Therapy, 2*, 1-15.

26. Charlton RS & Quatman, T (1999). A therapist's guide to the physiology of sexual response. In RS Charlton & ID Yalom (Eds.), *Treating sexual disorders* (pp.29-58). San Francisco, CA: Jossey-Bass Pub.

27. Fossa SD, Woehre H, Kurth KH, Hetherington J, Bakke H, Rustad DA, et al. (1997). Influence of urological morbidity on quality of life in patients with prostate cancer. *European Urology, 31*(Suppl.3), 3-8.

28. Thaler-DeMers D (2001). Intimacy issues: Sexuality, fertility, and relationships. *Seminars in Oncology Nursing, 17*, 255-262.

29. Schover LR (1997). *Sexuality and Fertility after Cancer*. New York: John Wiley and Sons, Inc.

30. Hughes MK (1996). Sexuality changes in the cancer patient: M.D. Anderson case reports and review. *Nurs Interven Oncol, 8*, 15-18.

31. Maurice, WL (1999). *Sexual medicine in primary care*. St. Louis, MO: Mosby.

32. Weeks GR & Gambescia N (2000). *Erectile dysfunction: Integrating couple therapy, sex therapy, and medical treatment*. New York: W.W. Norton & Co.

Strategies for Giving Bad News

Introduction

As oncologists, you must repeatedly give bad news over the course of a day; likely you will do it thousands of times over a long career. How to communicate bad news to patients, how to handle the difficult questions about their shortened survival and, how to respond to patients' anger or tears are challenging issues. Being able to communicate information clearly, and in a kind and sensitive manner and to listen empathically is the hallmark of the good physician. This chapter provides an approach to effective communication which is simple and readily applied.

Giving Bad News

Giving bad news which has the potential to drastically change a patient's life and future is best approached in several steps, which can be remembered by the acronym: S-P-I-K-E-S.

Table 8.1   S-P-I-K-E-S[1]

Setting up the Interview
- Review the chart and reflect on the information you must give. Choose a quiet room where you will not be interrupted and put your pager and beeper on silent.
- Invite the patient to include a family member, or more than one, if wanted.
- Sit down so that the patient and you are at eye level to dampen the "white coat syndrome."

Perception
- Find out the patient's current understanding of the illness and test results. In this way you will learn how much of an information gap there is between the actual medical facts and what the patient understands or believes.
- A simple statement: "Before I tell you the results of the test...I'd like to make sure that we are both on the same page. Would you tell me what you understand right now about your illness?"

Invitation
- This step avoids giving too much information too fast.
- Ask, "Is it OK if I go ahead and discuss what the findings were?" This may be especially important when a family member is present, and the patient may not want the relative to hear the information.
- Some patients (especially when the disease is advanced) may want much less detailed information at this juncture.

© 2000 by Walter F. Baile, MD[1]   (continued, next page)

Table 8.1   S-P-I-K-E-S (continued)[1]

Knowledge

- It is best to prepare the patient by making an empathic statement such as, "I'm afraid I have bad news for you." This avoids the patient being taken by surprise. The information should then be given in clear language without jargon to avoid misunderstandings.
- Remember that you can never make bad news better than it is and attempts to do so with false reassurance or by withholding information may result later in loss of trust.
- However, the information should be given in as kind, sympathetic and empathic manner as possible, at times touching the person's hand when it feels appropriate. This is often felt as expression of your concern.
- Equally important is to avoid unnecessarily frightening statements.

Emotions

- When news is very bad or unexpected, patients may express a range of emotions from shock to tears to anger.
- It is important to be patient and tolerate whatever the emotion is. If there are tears, move closer and offer a tissue. Several statements may help: "I can see that you did not expect this..." or "You know, you had a perfect right to believe that things were going well and this comes as a shock." or "Can you tell me how you are feeling?" (To family members, "Do you have thoughts about this?").
- These strategies often prevent escalation of the emotion and are appreciated by the patient and lead to the sense that, "The doctor cares about me *as a person*."
- When the statement is coupled with "This may be rough, but we'll get through it together," it also reassures the patient about your commitment to his/her continued care, irrespective of change in treatment plan.

Strategy and **S**ummary

- Having a strategy provides a roadmap for the patient and helps to reduce the significant anxiety associated with the uncertainty about the illness and the future.
- Patients should be encouraged to bring a family member or significant other, who can fill in the gaps in information which the patient may not hear due to anxiety.
- Concerns about the effect of the news on the family should be addressed. "I am worried about telling my children" is an issue that should always be addressed.
- It is crucial that bad news never be given without following up by describing the treatment plan you recommend.
- There is *never* a time to say, "There is nothing more I can do for you."

© 2000 by Walter F. Baile, MD[1]

Table 8.2   Difficult Questions May Arise in the Course of Giving Bad News

"Tell me, doctor, how bad is it?"
- Explore the question further by asking the patient exactly what he/she would like to know.
- Many patients have milestones they would like to meet (such as a trip they want to take) and want to know if they could go ahead with it. Others want to be able to plan for the future.
- When patients press for information about survival, it is best to give a range of possible time, accompanied by a hopeful statement: "While we're talking about a few months or maybe a year, we can hope that you will be one of those patients that live longer. Remember, you are a statistic of one."

"Isn't there anything more you can do?"
- When curative treatment must change to palliative, this especially may come up.
- It is usually a reaction of shock in a patient (even those who may have been expecting it)!
- Resist the temptation to offer another anti-cancer therapy which may diminish the patient's quality of life without much benefit.
- Instead make an empathic statement such as, "I wish there were another treatment that would not do you more harm than good right now." This communicates that you care about the patient's quality of life as well as prolonging life.

"I want a second opinion"
- Don't argue with the patient that another physician will come to the same conclusion as you.
- Some patients need time to come to grips with the implications of the bad news.

"The family says..."
- "You can't tell my father his cancer will come back. It will kill him."
- Resist the temptation to tell them you are ethically bound to tell the patient. Instead explore the relative's concerns by asking them to be more specific about what they are worried about.
- Often family members project their own anxieties onto the patient. Acknowledge their desire to protect the patient but suggest they, the patient and you speak together.
- If the patient truly wants to receive information only for the family, this should be respected.

When the patient presents for the first time with a metastatic or very advanced disease...
- Resist the temptation to raise the patient's expectations ("I'm going to make you the poster boy for lung cancer.") or to be too dismal ("There's nothing more we can do for you.").
- Employ the strategy of "hoping for the best and preparing for the worst."
- "You know I'm sorry to say that you do have very bad disease but I can assure you that we will give you the best treatment available and we can hope that things turn out better than would otherwise normally be the case."

Summary

Giving bad news is stressful for the patient, the family and the doctor. Communicating in ways in which patients feel emotionally supported increases their feeling of trust, hope, a sense of being respected as a person, and it promotes their willingness to be a partner with the doctor to achieve the best outcome possible.

Supporting Parents with Cancer: Screening and Psycho-education

Introduction

The National Cancer Institute estimates that twenty-four percent of adults with cancer, and one third of patients with breast cancer are parenting children under 18 years old. These patients experience their parenting role as a central to their identity, and may make treatment decisions with their children in mind.[3,4] Parental cancer can also produce significant distress for the children,[5] especially near the end of life.[6] Clinicians can enhance their alliance with patients and families, and help patients cope better with their illness when they recognize this aspect of the patients' lives.

Table 8.3   Screening: Get to Know the Children Through the Parent's Eyes

"Do you have children at home? Tell me about their personalities..."	• Parents usually talk readily about their children's pre-morbid temperaments and coping styles, and experience it as a welcome respite from the distress around their illness.
	• Eliciting a three dimensional picture of the children and the family life before the illness builds trust and demonstrates the clinician's interest in them as people separate from the illness.
" What have you told them about your illness? What words did you use?"	This sets the platform from which to begin the intervention around communication with children.
"How are they coping? What are your greatest concerns about your children?"	This allows you to address what is most pressing from the patient's perspective.
"Who would you talk with if you have concerns about your children?"	This allows you to share information about hospital or community-based resources for children's mental health.

Table 8.4   Education for Parents: Facilitate Honest Parent-child Communication

Euphemisms lead to confusion.
• Parents need to name the illness, i.e. use the real name "breast cancer" or "lymphoma," not euphemisms such as "lump" or "boo-boo" which can lead to confusion about everyday childhood illnesses being as serious as cancer.

"Protection" from the illness may be experienced by children as exclusion.
• Parents' natural desire to protect their children from distress is often an error of kindness that results in children feeling excluded from important family experiences, or worrying that the reality is so terrible that it cannot be talked about with their parents.
• The worst way for children to hear news about a parent's illness is to overhear it. This is inevitable if there has not been an open discussion.
• Children are usually more aware of what goes on around them than parents realize.

Welcome all questions warmly, find out what children are really asking about, and encourage children not to worry alone.
• Parents need to figure out what the child is really asking about by inquiring, "What got you thinking about that?"
• The real question is often quite specific and easier to answer than the imagined one.
• Questions do not always have to have immediate answers. Parents can validate the importance of a question and say that they need to think about it, or ask the doctor or other parent about it. Then they need to return to the child with a reasonable answer.
• Children must also be encouraged to bring back what they hear about their parent's illness from others, so that misinformation can be corrected, and support and reassurance can be given to the child.

Respect a child's wish not to talk.
• Children cannot be forced to talk about a parent's illness. Children who are not verbally expressive in general are unlikely to become big talkers about a parent's illness.
• All children need informational "news bulletins" throughout the course of the illness.
• Parents need to adjust their expectations and recognize that children need to hear directly about what is happening, but may not want to discuss it.

"What if my child asks if I am going to die?" (the question most feared by parents)
• Anticipating this with parents can allow them to feel freer about communicating with their children, and help them find an answer they are comfortable with.
• In most situations, parents can be joined in hoping for the best, and preparing for the worst. "Cancer can sometimes kill people, but I am doing everything I can to fight it and live as long as I can, as best as I can."
• Uncertainty is the hardest part for everyone involved. Parents can acknowledge this in the context of having a plan to produce the best possible outcome.

Table 8.4   Education for Parents: Hospital Visits

A child who wants to visit should usually be allowed to do so.	Exceptions to this would be an agitated, delirious parent who might be frightening to a child. In these cases, it is best to wait until the parent's mental status is improved or sedated, so that a child can have a quiet visit, even if it is talking to or holding the hand of a sleeping parent.
Prepare the child for what they will see and hear.	Describe in advance what or whom the child will see in the hospital, medical technology, the parent's mental status, what they will be able to do or touch in the room.
Explore and alleviate specific fears.	Children may express fears of seeing blood, or of seeing their parent receive an injection or have a medical crisis while they are present.
Bring a designated support person.	• The child should dictate the length of the visit. • Have them accompanied by a familiar adult who will be able to leave whenever the child is ready.
De-brief after the visit.	• Talk with the child about what was best, worst, or most surprising about the visit. • Support whatever kind of visit the child was able to have.
If a visit is not possible, support other methods of communication.	Children can send cards, drawings, photos, and hear from others about the pleasure that these items bring their ill parent.

Each normal developmental stage builds on the previous one. Coping strategies and parenting guidelines that are helpful for the youngest children, may also help older ones and adults.

Table 8.5   Education for Parents: Developmental Guidelines

Infants & Toddlers (under 3 years) are working on tasks of attachment and attunement with caregivers.	• Maintain consistency in their immediate environment (portacrib, toys, foods) and a few regular caregivers. • Provide regular brief contact with the ill parent except if delirious. • Photos, letters, memories from others can help to tell the story later.
Pre-schoolers (3-6 years old) are egocentric, use associative logic and magical thinking. (continued, next page)	• Explore the child's understanding and fantasies about the illness and its causes, dispel guilt or personal responsibility for the illness. • Explore specific questions the child has about death and difficulty grasping its permanence (this is developmentally appropriate). • Be prepared for concrete, disarming questions about illness and death, and disconnection of content and emotion.

Table 8.5   Education for Parents: Developmental Guidelines (continued)

School-age Children (7 - 12 years) are mastering skills and rules, and are focussed on friends and activities.	• Provide direct explanations about the illness and it's treatment. Distinguish between effects of the illness, and side effects of treatment. Dispel misconceptions about contagion or causes of cancer. • Expect coping through doing and maintain as much normal activity as possible. • Designate an adult point-person (best friend's parent, neighbor) to make sure the child has assigned materials for school and extracurricular activities. • Find the best times for conversations. These are often not face-to-face, e.g. in the car, while cooking, etc.
Adolescents (13 - 21 years) are engaged in separation-individuation and may have developmentally normal ambivalent relationships with parents	• Respect established methods of coping: talking or not talking.· Support the love that exists despite conflict. • Normalize the value of non-parental adult support. • Identify high-risk young people who are acting out, withdrawal, overcompensating. • Involve young adults in active decision-making about how geographically close or distant they want to be in the context of the parent's illness.

Referral Guidelines

Coping with a parental medical illness is stressful in any family. Most parents and children can get adequate support from family, community, and medical resources. In the setting of parental discord or divorce, however, providing for the needs of the children may be especially complicated. Clinicians need to be alert for conflict between parents that interferes with open communication with children, or the maintenance of their usual activities and function. Bridging this conflict in the service of the children may require referral for more intensive parent guidance, family therapy, or even engaging the Department of Social Services/Child Welfare or the courts through a Guardian *ad Litem*.

Adults and children may be particularly vulnerable to mood disorders during the course of a medical illness in the family. Any parent or child with a prior history of mental illness or difficulty functioning may require additional mental health support. An ill parent who begins to talk about their children being better off without them or who shows signs of major depression should be referred for full psychiatric evaluation. The well spouse who is having trouble coping may also benefit from individual counseling that will ultimately serve the interests of the entire family. Refer for evaluation by a child mental health specialist children who exhibit persistent difficulties in two out of the three areas of function (school, family, peers), or children who exhibit any signs of depression or suicidal ideation.

Spiritual/Religious Communication with Patients and Families

Introduction

Brief guidelines for spiritual care are part of the NCCN clinical practice distress management guidelines, with the goal that the primary oncology team will be able to identify the patient whose distress is related to a spiritual or religious issue, and to refer the patient to an appropriate clergy, chaplain, or pastoral counselor.[13]

Be familiar with the pastoral resources in your hospital and community. It is helpful to have an informal relationship with a representative from the major faiths of patients in your practice so that when questions arise that relate to a particular religious ritual or practice, you can call for informal advice about how to handle it. Clinicians can become comfortable communicating with patients and families about spiritual or religious issues.

Table 8.6   Key Reasons Spiritual Issues are Important to Patients with Cancer

- Serious illness may create a "spiritual crisis" in which long-held beliefs are challenged and result in significant distress (e.g. loss of faith, feeling of being punished).
- Beliefs may be playing a major role in how the patient is coping with illness.
- Religious beliefs may affect decisions to accept or reject a doctor's recommendations for treatment (e.g. refusal of transfusions, continuation of life supports).
- Some patients and families want to discuss these issues with the doctor, particularly as illness progresses and when death is near.[14,15,16]

Assessment

It is best to have a standard spiritual question or two to ask that is compatible with your manner of taking a clinical history, with the goal to determine whether there are pertinent religious issues affecting coping or treatment decisions:

Table 8.7   Questions for Information on Spiritual Attitudes

- Do you have some beliefs that have helped you cope with difficult things in the past? Were they religious or spiritual beliefs? Are they important to you now in coping with illness?"
- Are any of your beliefs causing you distress in coping with illness? Any conflict between your beliefs and the treatments recommended?
- Are there any religious practices that you need help to continue during illness (e.g. special foods, prayers)?
- For a formal tool for spiritual and religious assessment (cf. Chapter 2, Figure 2.8).

Table 8.8   Frequent Problems of Patients Referred for Pastoral Counseling

- Dealing with anticipated or current grief in patient and family ("How can I face the loss?")
- Beliefs that are challenged by illness ("God has forsaken me.")
- Concerns and need to discuss death and concepts of afterlife ("What is out there?")
- Loss of faith ("I no longer can believe as I did before.")
- Desire for prayer or other rituals ("I need to ask for help in coping.")
- Loss of hope ("I have no hope for the future.") - Hopelessness may be a cardinal symptom of depression/suicidal ideation and may need to be evaluated by a mental health professional.
- Loss of meaning in life ("I cannot find meaning to life since I am ill.")
- Dealing with guilt from past ("God is punishing me.")
- Treatments recommended are in conflict with deep held religious beliefs ("I cannot accept the doctor's recommendation because it is against my religion.")
- Persons who have lost contact with their former religious community and who wish assistance in the absence of their community ties

Boundaries

Be clear that you have respect for the beliefs and practices of each patient, without regard to your own. It is not appropriate for a physician to initiate prayer with the patient, however, an exception might be in the situation where the physician and patient are from the same religious community, and the doctor feels comfortable in doing so.

References

Strategies for Giving Bad News

1. Baile WF, Buckman R, Lenzi R, Glober G, Beale EA & Kudelka AP (2000). SPIKES-A six-step protocol for delivering bad news: Application to the patient with cancer. *The Oncologist*, 5, 302-311.

2. Buckman R & Baile WF (2001). "A Practical Guide to Communication Skills in Cancer Care" (3-set CD-ROM). Medical Audio-Visual Communications.

Supporting Parents with Cancer

3. Duric V, Stockler, M. (2001). Patients preferences for adjuvant chemotherapy in early breast cancer: a review of what makes it worthwhile. *Lancet Oncology*, 2, 691-697.

4. Yellen SB, Cella DF. (1995). Someone to live for: social well-being, parenthood status, and decision-making in oncology. *Journal of Clinical Oncology*, 13(5), 1255-64.

5. Compas BE, Worsham NL, Epping-Jordan JE, Grant KE, Mireault G, Howell DC, Malcarne VL. (1994). When mom or dad has cancer: markers of psychological distress in cancer patients, spouses, and children. *Health Psychology, 13(6),* 507-15.

6. Siegel K, Mesagno FP, Karus D, Christ G, Banks K, Moynihan R. (1992). Psychosocial Adjustment of Children with a Terminally Ill Parent. *Journal of the American Academy of Child and Adolescent Psychiatry, 31(2),* 327-333.

Suggested Reading for Parents:

7. Harpham WS (1997). *When a parent has cancer: A guide to caring for your children.* New York: Harper Collins.

8. Heiney SP, Hermann JF, Bruss KV & Fincannon JL (2001). *Cancer in the family: Helping children cope with a parent's illness.* Oklahoma City, OK: American Cancer Society.

9. McCue K & Bonn R (1994). *How to help children through a parent's serious illness.* New York: St. Martin's Griffin.

Suggested Reading for Clinicians:

10. Muriel AC & Rauch PK (2003). Suggestions for patients on how to talk with children about a parent's cancer. *Journal of Supportive Oncology, 1,* 143-145.

11. Rauch PK, Muriel AC & Cassem NH (2002). Parents with cancer: Who's looking after the children? *Journal of Clinical Oncology, 20,* 4399-402.

12. Rauch PK & Muriel AC (2004). The importance of parenting concerns among patients with cancer. *Critical Reviews in Oncology/ Hematology, 49,* 37-42.

Spiritual/Religious Communication with Patients and Families

13. NCCN 1.2005 Distress Management, *The Complete Library of NCCN Clinical Practice Guidelines in Oncology [CD-Rom].* Jenkintown, Pennsylvania: ©National Comprehensive Cancer Network, May 2005. To view the most recent and complete version of the guidelines, go online to www.nccn.org.

14. Handzo G & Koenig H (2004). Spiritual care: Whose job is it anyway? *Southern Medical Journal, 97,* 1242-1244.

15. Ehman JW, Ott BB, Short TH, Ciampa RC & Hansen-Flaschen J (1999). Do patients want physician to inquire about their spiritual or religious beliefs if they become gravely ill? *Archives of Internal Medicine, 5,* 16-18.

16. McCord G, Gilchrist VJ, Grossman SD, King BD, McCormick KF, Oprandi AM, et al. (2004). Discussing spirituality with patients: A rational and ethical approach. *Annals of Family Medicine, 2,* 356-361.

Brain Cancer

The psychiatric effects of primary and metastatic brain tumors present challenges for patients, caregivers, and clinicians. The emotional burden is considerable. It is unclear whether the neuropsychiatric sequelae of primary and metastatic brain tumors are distinctly different. From a clinical standpoint, they both result from brain injury.

Table 9.1   Incidence and Prognosis of Brain Tumors

Cancer in the central nervous system (CNS), and its treatment, can be expected to affect cognition, mood, and personality. Loss of the patient's independence and identity means more responsibility and stress for caregivers of these patients than for caregivers of other cancer patients.[1]

CNS tumors that are usually, though not always, benign (i.e., *meningiomas, craniopharyngiomas*) can cause significant neuropsychiatric and emotional morbidity because of mass effect, disruption of endocrine function, and recurrence.

Primary malignant brain tumors - most difficult malignancies to treat; poor prognoses. Overall five-year survival rates approaching 33%[2]

Gliomas - most common primary brain tumors, accounting for > 40% of all new cases[3]

Metastatic brain tumors indicate advancing disease; often an ominous sign. Over 150,000 new cases of metastatic brain tumors develop each year, accounting for 80-90% of all new cases of CNS cancer annually.

These primary tumors account for 85% of metastases to the brain:
• Lung (esp. small cell and adenocarcinoma)
• Breast   • Melanoma
• Renal cell   • Colon[4,5]

Patients with *leptomeningeal* metastasis are likely to develop diffuse neurological deficits (included slowed cognition) and usually require treatment associated with neuropsychiatric side effects (i.e., brain radiation, intrathecal chemotherapy).

Leptomeningeal spread of cancer occurs in 5% of patients with systemic cancers, including solid tumors, especially:
• Lung cancer   • Breast cancer
• Melanoma   • Lymphomas and leukemias[6]

Table 9.2   Brain Tumor Characteristics that Affect Cognitive Function

Occur in 70% of cases of CNS malignancy.
 Factors of importance

• *Location of lesion*	• *Dominant hemisphere lesions* (or effects of their treatment) may be associated with loss of verbal or written language function.
	• *Non-dominant hemisphere* disease may be associated with impairment of visual-spatial processing ability.
	• *Frontal and temporal* lesions of either hemisphere can cause memory dysfunction.
	• More *posterior* located disease may be associated with inability to process visual cues resulting in various agnosias.[7]
• *Rate of tumor growth*	• Rapidly growing tumors are more likely to cause acute altered mental status (e.g., delirium) or sudden loss of cognitive ability.
	• Slow growing benign or malignant tumors are likely to cause insidious changes of cognition, consistent with early stages of primary dementias.
• *Number of tumor foci*	• Multiple tumor foci increase the likelihood of involvement of critical CNS structures or neurotransmitter pathways.
• *Patient age*	• Elderly patients and patients with pre-morbid cognitive impairment may have diminished cognitive reserve at baseline and are thus more vulnerable to new or progressing CNS insults than younger or very high functioning patients.
• *Secondary effects of tumor and treatment*	• Anatomic damage may be caused by surgery or radiation therapy.
• *Diaschisis effects*	• Lesions can cause focal dysfunction in anatomically separate areas of the brain via disruption of connected fiber tracts.
Frontal Lobe Syndromes (continued, next page)	• Descriptions of prefrontal syndromes are relevant to problems routinely associated with treatment of CNS cancer.[8]
	• Distant pathology can cause presentations identical to syndromes associated with frontal lesions.
	• Mixed presentations should be expected.
	• Compromised higher executive function. *Dysexecutive syndrome* (most common) - psychomotor slowing. Patients perseverate, lose ability to switch cognitive sets, and have difficulty taking on new tasks. They may develop diminished attention to self-care and flattening of affect. Quite often they appear to be depressed. The constellation of symptoms also suggests progression of subcortical dementia.

Table 9.2   Brain Tumor Characteristics that Affect Cognitive Function (continued)

Frontal Lobe Syndromes (continued)	• *Disinhibited type syndrome* - emotional labile, poor social judgment, and little insight • *Apathetic syndrome* - verbal and motor slowing, and eventually urinary incontinence, and lower extremity weakness[8]
Temporal Lobe Tumors	• Function of direct damage to dominant/non-dominant sites resulting in deficits described above and physical or physiological disruption of neurotransmitter pathways to and from the frontal lobes • Can also result in frontal/pre-frontal lobe syndromes characteristic of damage to anterior structures

Table 9.3   Brain Tumors - Effects on Personality, Mood, Psychosis, Disinhibition

Changes in personality	• Presentations consistent with almost all primary psychiatric disorders have been described in patients with primary and malignant brain tumors. • Rare neuropsychiatric syndromes also come in all forms. • At first glance without examination and work-up, there is little if anything that distinguishes psychopathology due to brain tumors. • Often associated with frontal lobe (up to 70%) and temporal lobe (>50%) tumors and may be the first sign of an occult carcinoma, e.g. in lung cancer. • Often the presentation involves "coarsening" or exaggeration of pre-morbid personality traits. • Changes are usually subtle in early on and become more pronounced with disease progression. • There may be marked, fairly dramatic change that brings the patient to evaluation.
Depression	• Incidence of 25 - 30% has been found in ambulatory settings using strict criteria, and much higher estimates has been found in peri-operative populations.[9,10] • Mood disorders including depression and mania have commonly been associated with frontal and temporal lobe lesions. • Again, because of diaschesis, tumors in other locations could easily cause the same presentations. • Pituitary tumors (e.g., craniopharyngiomas) may render a patient hormone-dependent with effects on mood, libido, and fatigue. • Drug side effects, notably those of corticosteroids and anticonvulsants, are common causes of mood disorders in this setting. • "Reactive depressions" in patients trying to cope with loss of independence, cognitive ability, physical function, and disease poorly responsive to treatment are to be expected.

(continued, next page)

Table 9.3   Brain Tumors - Effects on Personality, Mood, Psychosis, Disinhibition (continued)

Anxiety	• Anxiety and "schizophrenia" have traditionally been associated with temporal lobe tumors. Anxiety is probably more common.
Psychosis	• Hallucinations and/or delusions can be a function of delirium, seizure and drug side effects.
Disinhibition	• Presents as paroxysmal rage or sudden violence and impulsivity. • May require environmental changes, anti-psychotics, or mood stabilizers to protect the patient and others. • These behaviors typically resolve gradually with disease progression.

Table 9.4   Adverse Effects of Cancer Therapy

Radiation Therapy- (XRT) is integral to management of known primary and metastatic CNS tumors, and as prophylaxis against leptomeningeal metastasis to the CNS. Brain XRT is associated with three major neurotoxicity syndromes.[11]	• *Acute radiation syndrome-* occurs during or shortly after completion of XRT; characterized by delirium, nausea and vomiting. It is thought to be associated with cerebral edema and raised intracranial pressure. Patients undergoing cranial XRT are usually treated with corticosteroids to prevent or minimize raised intracranial pressure and so the acute radiation syndrome is infrequently encountered.
	• *Early delayed radiation syndrome-* due to temporary demyelination and is characterized by reemergence of neurological symptoms and sometimes a "somnolence syndrome." It usually resolves over days or weeks and again, steroids are protective.
	• *Late delayed radiation syndrome* develops months or years after completion of XRT and involves progressive, often irreversible cognitive impairment. Radiation necrosis and progressive leukoencephalopathy are implicated as primary causes of the late delayed syndrome.
	• Several other XRT-associated disorders of cognitive function have been described in children and adults.[12]
	• Factors that influence XRT-induced neurotoxicity include:
	  • age • cumulative radiation dose
	  • concomitant chemotherapy • length of survival post-XRT[11]

Chemotherapy- blood brain barrier prevents passage of many chemotherapy and other antineoplastic agents into the CNS. (continued, next page)	• Several antineoplastic drugs are associated with neuropsychiatric side effects when delivered to the CNS by intravenous or intrathecal routes. • Acute encephalopathy is seen with administration of methotrexate, which may also cause a permanent leukoencephalopathy. • Cytosine arabinoside is associated with acute encephalopathy, which usually resolves, and cerebellar syndrome, which may resolve or persist indefinitely.

Table 9.4   Adverse Effects of Cancer Therapy (continued)

Chemotherapy (continued)	• The interferons are associated with variable degrees of cognitive dysfunction. • Procarbazine is a weak monoamine oxidase inhibitor which occasionally causes anxiety and must be used cautiously, if at all with most anti-psychotic and antidepressant drugs.[13]
Surgery- resection of primary and metastatic brain tumors often tolerated remarkably well	• Peri-operative delirium is common. • Patients with lesions in sensitive areas may experience temporary (sometimes permanent) language or motor deficits that result in problematic anxiety and depression.
Corticosteroids, Analgesics, Anticonvulsants	• *Steroids* are generally protective against vasogenic edema and raised intracranial pressure. The drugs can cause psychosis, mania, and especially with longterm use, depressive symptoms. Dose decrease or discontinuation is often helpful. When that is not possible, symptomatic treatment with psychotropic medications is appropriate. • More vulnerable to sedating effects of *opioid analgesics*. • Anticonvulsants, especially but not exclusively older drugs including *phenobarbital, phenytoin* (Dilantin®), and *carbamazepine* (Tegretol®), may cause sedation and confusion at therapeutic or high levels.

Table 9.5   Assessment

• Primary or reactive mood, anxiety, and thought disorders overlap with those caused by tumor or treatment.
• Patients are often poor historians.
• Evaluation process is fairly straightforward, if not always revealing.
• Thorough history should be obtained with attention to premorbid symptomatology.
• Especially in cases of cognitive impairment- rely on family members or other caregivers for aspects of the history.
• Because of the great emotional and prognostic significance of cancer in the nervous system, it is important to ask anxious and depressed patients about reactions to diagnosis, understanding of clinical status, and perceptions of the future.
• A search for reversible and treatable causes of symptoms should be commenced, including review of medications as well as laboratory, electrophysiological, and neuroimaging studies.
• *Neuropsychological assessment* is invaluable in evaluation of the brain tumor patient with behavioral symptoms.[7] In early stages of disease, neuropsychological test batteries can detect and characterize subtle cognitive deficits. Serial tests help track rate of recovery or decline. Characterization of impairment (deficit vs. handicap) is useful for post-treatment rehabilitation and mobilization of appropriate support resources.[7]

Table 9.6   Pharmacological Treatments

Few data are available from clinical trials to guide use of psychotropic drugs in patients with brain tumors.	• Guidelines for use of antidepressants, anxiolytics, and antipsychotics in cancer patients are applicable (cf. Chapter 4). • The general recommendation to "start low and go slow" is especially applicable to treatment of patients with cancer in the CNS. • *Antidepressants- Tricyclic antidepressants* may not be well tolerated because of sedative and anticholinergic effects. Use of *bupropion* (Wellbutrin®) is not recommended in any patient with past history of seizures or current seizure risk. Drug-drug interactions should be considered. Concomitant use of selective serotonin reuptake inhibitors and some anticonvulants (i.e., *carbamazepine* (Tegretol®), *phenytoin* (Dilantin®) can increase levels of the latter. • *Anxiolytics* - Use in patients sensitive to sedative effects of benzodiazepines. The use of shorter half-life drugs such as *alprazolam* (Xanax®) and *lorazepam* (Ativan®) is preferred. This drug class may also cause disinhibition or agitation in patients with significant cognitive impairment. In such cases low dose antipsychotics may be used for the same purpose. *Buspirone* (Buspar®) metabolism may be altered by some anticonvulsants.
Antipsychotics	• Many if not all patients with CNS disease are on anticonvulsants, so the hypothetical problem of lowered seizure threshold from a phenothiazine and butyrophenone antipsychotics is minimized. • Newer atypical antipsychotics, e.g., *quetiapine* (Seroquel®) and *olanzapine* (Zyprexa®), have been associated with hyperglycemia; attention to serum glucose levels is appropriate, especially in patients treated with corticosteroids.
Psychostimulants	• *methylphenidate* (Ritalin®), d-amphetamine, and possibly *modafinil* (Provigil®) very effective in palliation of psychomotor slowing, depression, and cognitive impairment associated with treatment of brain tumors.[14] Generally well tolerated, but can cause anxiety and insomnia and are problematic in patients with unstable blood pressure.

Table 9.7   Non-pharmacological Treatments

| Psychotherapy | • Supportive, using crisis intervention and psychoeducational techniques[2]
• Primary goal to provide accurate information, and decrease uncertainty and fear to the degree possible
• Relaxation training for patients without major cognitive impairment
• Support groups
• National advocacy organizations such as the National Brain Tumor Foundation, http://www.braintumor.org, and the American Brain Tumor Association, http://abta.org, can provide other valuable resources for the supportive care of patients with CNS cancer. |
| (continued, next page) | |

Table 9.7   Non-pharmacological Treatments (continued)

Cognitive and Vocational Rehabilitation	• Neuropsychological and vocational testing can identify remediable deficits and help patients and caregivers to develop realistic goals regarding education, employment, independence and safety in the home.[7]
Support for families and caregivers	• Families and caregivers of patients with cancer in the nervous system face all the problems of families of patients with non-neurological cancer and often the added burden of dealing with progressive cognitive decline and poor prognosis.[2] Rates of psychiatric morbidity are higher in caregivers than in the general population. Ongoing medical and psychosocial care of the patient with CNS cancer should include assessment of caregiver support. Families and caregivers can benefit from many of the supportive techniques used to help patients. Support groups and education can be especially helpful. In some cases it may be necessary to identify or provide resources for individual therapy or pharmacotherapy for depression.

Breast Cancer

Breast cancer is the most common cancer in women and is second only to lung cancer in cancer deaths in women. Over 200,000 women in the United States are diagnosed yearly, and over 40,000 women will die. Although more than 85% of women diagnosed with Stage I breast cancer will be alive in 5 years, survival drops dramatically when cancers are diagnosed at later stages. A woman's ability to manage a breast cancer diagnosis and treatment commonly changes over the course of illness and depends on medical, psychological and social factors.[15,16]

Evaluation

Table 9.8   Factors Affecting Adjustment to Diagnosis and Treatment

- The disease itself (stage at diagnosis, type of treatments recommended, symptoms, clinical course and prognosis).
- Prior level of adjustment, patient's own personality and coping style and prior experience with loss
- The threat that breast cancer poses to attaining age appropriate development goals (e.g., marriage, pregnancy, child rearing, career, retirement)
- Cultural, spiritual and religious attitudes
- Presence of emotionally supportive persons
- Potential for physical and psychological rehabilitation

Many women adapt well to learning the diagnosis and to the treatments offered with the support offered by oncologists, nurses, social workers and the clergy and do not require psychiatric support. Some women should be referred for psychiatric consultation.

Table 9.9   Reasons for Psychiatric Consult

Urgent Psychiatric Consult ***Current Symptoms/History of:***	**Consider Psychiatric Consult** ***Facing Difficult Decisions:***
• Depression and anxiety • Suicidal thinking (attempt) • Substance or alcohol abuse • Confusional state (delirium or encephalopathy) • Mood swings, insomnia, or irritability from steroids • Paralyzed by cancer treatment decisions • Fear death during surgery or terrified by loss of control under anesthesia • Request euthanasia • Seem unable to provide informed consent • Very old, young, pregnant, nursing, single, or alone • Adjusting to multiple losses • Managing multiple life stresses	• How to deal with family history of breast cancer • Whether to undergo genetic testing • Whether to inform family of results of genetic testing • Whether to have risk-reducing surgery such as prophylactic mastectomy and/or prophylactic oophorectomy after a cancer diagnosis or if BRCA 1 or 2 mutation carrier • Whether to have mastectomy or limited resection followed by irradiation • Whether to have breast reconstruction following mastectomy • If having reconstruction, which natural tissue or implant to select • If pregnant at the time of diagnosis, whether to terminate the pregnancy to protect the fetus from teratogenic effects of alkylating agents • Whether to attempt pregnancy after breast cancer treatment (concern about dangerousness for mother) • Whether to adopt a child given uncertainty of future • Whether or when to tell employer, colleagues, friends, new relationship/sexual partner about current breast cancer treatment or cancer history • How to tell children in developmentally appropriate language about diagnosis or need for absences from home for surgery

Although only 5% of breast cancer occurs in women younger than 40 years of age, a disproportionately large number of these women seek psychiatric consultation.

Table 9.10 Issues Especially Relevant to Younger Breast Cancer Patients

• Sexual side-effects of treatments • Fertility and child rearing • Self and body image	• Genetic testing[17] • Education, career • Relationships, children	• Prophylactic mastectomy or oophorectomy

The hereditary breast cancer syndrome accounts for only 5% – 7% of all breast cancer cases. In some cancer centers, psychiatric consultation is an essential part of the evaluation process of the women who considers prophylactic mastectomy or prophylactic oophorectomy as risk reducing surgery, after testing positive for a germ-line mutation in BRCA1 and BRCA2 genes.

Table 9.11 Components of the Psychiatric Evaluation of Women who Consider Prophylactic Mastectomy and/or Prophylactic Oophorectomy

- Family cancer history[18]
- Personal history of breast, ovarian cancer and other cancers
- Psychiatric history
  - Anxiety disorder
  - Depressive disorder
  - Body dysmorphic disorder
  - Personality disorder
- Perception of cancer risk and anxiety associated with perceptions
- Understanding of actual risk
- Satisfaction with previous plastic surgeries
- Litigation history
- History of abuse, rape or assault
- Sexual, pregnancy and breast feeding history
- Desire to have (more) children
- Timing of prophylactic mastectomy or oophorectomy relative to planned pregnancies
- Feasibility of childrearing with uncertainty about the future
- Partner's role in the consideration of prophylactic surgery
- Strategies to reduce anxiety offered, regardless of the patient's decision

Table 9.12 Burdens of the Patient's Partner/Husband

- Facing uncertainty (death) and loss of control
- Participating in many doctor appointments, care
- Continuing work; managing diminished finances
- Managing additional responsibility, such as child rearing, domestic responsibilities
- Adjusting to altered appearance and temporary (or permanent) loss of sexual partner
- Caring for a (sometimes) ungrateful, irritable, depressed partner

Interventions

The interventions for women with breast cancer include drugs, psychotherapy, specialized programs and complimentary treatments.

Table 9.13 Pharmacological Interventions for Breast Cancer Patients*

Pre-surgery, pre and post chemotherapy, anxiety/agitation	Anxiolytics - *lorazepam* (Ativan®), *alprazolam* (Xanax®), *clonazepam* (Klonopin®)
Antiemetics pre- and post-chemotherapy	*lorazepam* (Ativan®), *alprazolam* (Xanax®)

(continued, next page)

* Cf. Chapter 4.

Table 9.13 Pharmacological Interventions for Breast Cancer Patients (continued)*

Insomnia during any phase of cancer treatment	• Hypnotics - *zolpidem* (Ambien®), *eszopiclone* (Lunesta®) • Benzodiazepines - *temazepam* (Restoril®)
Depression, panic, generalized anxiety;	• Antidepressants - *sertraline* (Zoloft®), *paroxetine* (Paxil®), *duloxetine* (Cymbalta®), *escitalopram* (Lexapro®), *fluoxetine* (Prozac®), *citalopram* (Celexa®)
Vasomotor menopausal symptoms (hot flashes)	• Antidepressants - *sertraline* (Zoloft®), *paroxetine* (Paxil®),[19] *venlafaxine* (Effexor®)
Unrelenting fatigue after chemotherapy or irradiation	• Psychostimulants - *modafinil* (Provigil®), *methylphenidate* (Ritalin®)
Post-mastectomy neuropathic pain; peripheral neuropathy	• Tricyclic antidepressants - *nortriptyline* (Pamelor®), *amitriptyline* (Elavil®) • Antidepressants - *duloxetine* (Cymbalta®) • Anti-convulsants - *gabapentin* (Neurontin®) • Analgesics

* *Cf. Chapter 4.*

Table 9.14 Non-Pharmacological Interventions for Breast Cancer Patients*

Psychotherapy

Patients at all stages; those who need to make treatment decisions	• Individual Therapy - Exploratory, psychodynamic, supportive, cognitive and behavioral elements
Patients at time of diagnosis, with relapse or with metastatic disease	• Group Therapy - Supportive, cognitive, and behavioral elements

Specialized Programs

Appearance during chemotherapy	• Look Good . . . Feel Better® (www.lookgoodfeelbetter.org)
Sexual dysfunction	• Sexual counseling, rehabilitation
Lymphedema	• Physical therapy
Nutrition and avoiding weight gain	• Nutritional counseling
Fitting for appropriate prosthesis	• Prosthetic consultants

Complementary Treatments

Hot flashes	• Acupuncture
Chemotherapy or irradiation	• Gentle exercise and toning - Yoga, Pilates, Tai Chi

* *Cf. Chapter 5.*

Table 9.15 Interventions for Psychiatric Side Effects of Anti-estrogens[20,†*]

Irritability	• Antidepressants - *sertraline* (Zoloft®), *paroxetine* (Paxil®), *escitalopram* (Lexapro®), *fluoxetine* (Prozac®), *citalopram* (Celexa®) • Anxiolytics - *lorazepam* (Ativan®), *alprazolam* (Xanax®), *clonazepam* (Klonopin®)
Depression	• Antidepressants
Insomnia	• Hypnotics - *zolpidem* (Ambien®), *eszopiclone* (Lunesta®) • Benzodiazepines: *temazepam* (Restoril®)
Hot-flashes/ night-sweats	• Selective serotonin reuptake inhibitors (SSRI's) - *sertraline* (Zoloft®), *paroxetine* (Paxil®)[19] • Serotonin norepinephrine reuptake inhibitors (SNRI's®) - *venlafaxine* (Effexor®)
Weight gain	• Nutrition consult

† *Women who are eligible for antiestrogen therapy (tamoxifen, raloxifene, anastrazole, and exemestane) are treated for a period of years.*
* *Cf. Chapter 4.*

Table 9.16 Major Sexual Issues in Breast Cancer Patients*

• Decreased libido (desire)

• Decreased vaginal lubrication

• Painful sex

• Decreased pleasure in sex

• Embarrassment about drains, scars, implants, alopecia, lymphedema, weight gain or loss

• Concern partner will injure during sexual intercourse

* *Cf. Chapter 7, Sexual Dysfunction.*

Table 9.17 Benefits of Psychiatric/Group Intervention in Addressing Major Issues with Metastatic Breast Cancer

Issues	Benefits
• Fear of and adjustment to pain, physical and cognitive deterioration • Mourning the loss of autonomous function, old roles, hopes and aspirations • Altering, reducing and/or phasing out work and parenting commitments • Preparing children and other loved ones both emotionally and practically for death • Living with uncertainty of life span • Adapting to a series of treatments, knowing that treatment is offered without hope for cure • Managing life disruption due to many out-patient visits and hospitalizations • Fear of death • Considering practical issues about where to die, funeral or memorial services, bequeaths, etc.	• Opportunity to address existential, physical, emotional, social, psychosexual and relationship (family and others) concerns • Opportunity to express emotions, gain support, manage anxiety, fear, depression • Source of meaningful information • Challenge pessimistic thoughts • Consider priorities. • Manage treatment side effects (promote adherence to cancer treatment) • Phase specific issues (i.e., preparation for death)

Gastrointestinal Cancer

These cancers comprise a diverse group of neoplasms of the GI tract each with unique psychosocial issues and psychiatric complications. They have in common the GI tract as their organ system of origination. They have significant overlap in physical signs and symptoms referable to upper and lower tracts.

Table 9.18 Interventions for Common Problems in Esophageal and Gastric Cancer

Distress at extent and gravity of disease at diagnosis	• Provide consistent support. • Clearly outline a plan for treatment.
Preoccupation with anorexia, eating and weight	• Help patient cope with lower weight, loss of appetite. • Suggest several smaller meals and diet supplements. • Acknowledge that family support is critical, but also can be a source of conflict.

Social embarrassment of feeding tubes	• Ask what the feeding tube means to the patient.
	• Develop strategies for timing of feeding and preservation of social life.
	• Explore special clothing to conceal appliances.
	• For those who have trouble swallowing the following medications can be used (cf. Chapter 4):
	   • **For depression:** *mirtazepine* (Remeron®) sol tabs, *sertraline* (Zoloft®) liquid, *citalopram* (Celexa®) wafer;
	   • **For anxiety:** *clonazepam* (Klonopin®) wafers;
	   • **For restlessness:** *olanzapine* (Zyprexa®, Zydis®), *risperidone* (Risperdal®) m-tabs.

Social isolation and shame around regurgitation, belching, flatulence	• Validate feelings. • Suggest practical interventions such as support groups, simethicone.
History of alcohol and tobacco use (cf. protocols in Head and Neck Cancer section)	• Directly inquire about past history and active substance use. • Monitor for withdrawal syndromes from each. • Treat withdrawal and addiction as early as possible. • Suggest nicotine replacement for tobacco. • Benzodiazepines for alcohol withdrawal. • Assess other coping tools.
Fear of increasing pain	• Conduct a through pain assessment with each visit. • Treat pain aggressively. • Treat anxiety.

Table 9.19 Interventions for Common Problems in Colo-rectal Cancer

Guilt over delay in screen colonoscopy	• Use empathic listening. • Help patient focus on present care. • Encourage support group.
Variable adjustment to stoma/ostomy	• Assess coping of spouse/partner with demands of living with ostomy. • Enlist help for a Wound, Ostomy, Continence Nurse. • Encourage support groups (e.g. American Cancer Society). • Directly inquire about sexual functioning. • Consider *sildenafil* (Viagra®), *tadalafil* (Cialis®), *vardenafil* (Levitra®) for men with erectile dysfunction. • Suggest special clothing to conceal bags. • Suggest special bags to manage flatulence. • Suggest simethicone for flatulence. • Consult dietitian for diet management.
Burden of possible familial increased risk of colon cancer	• Allow patient to express guilt and other emotions openly. • Assist patient in ways to communicate risk to family members.
Anticipatory anxiety and social embarrassment about acute or chronic diarrhea and fecal incontinence	• Suggest anti-diarrheal medications. • Suggest stool softeners. • Emphasize regular irrigation of ostomy. • Antidepressants, benzodiazepines to treat recurrent anxiety and agoraphobia. • Suggest adult diapers. • Implement bowel training program for regularity.

Depression	• Antidepressants should be tailored for bowel function.
	  • Specific serotonin reuptake inhibitors can cause slightly looser stool.
	  • Tricyclic antidepressants and serotonin/ neuroepinephrine reuptake inhibitors such as *duloxetine* (Cymbalta®) and *venlafaxine* (Effexor®) are constipating.
	  • *Buproprion* (Wellbutrin®) is mildly constipating.

Delirium- most common with organ failure at end of life	• Manage most distressing aspects such as agitation and paranoid ideation with antipsychotics. • Explain medical basis of delirium to family. • Utilize strategies to minimize risk of delirium (watch anticholinergic side effects). • Reassess opioid regimen and consider rotating to another opioid. • Cf. Chapter 6, Cognitive Disorders.

Table 9.20 Interventions for Common Problems in Pancreatic Cancer

Depressive symptoms present at time of diagnosis, often with anxiety/restlessness	• Assess mood/anxiety at each visit. • Consider antidepressants early, particularly serotonin reuptake inhibitors. • Anti-anxiety medications to quell anxiety. • Cf. Chapter 6, Anxiety.
Feeling devastated at not being a surgical candidate for Whipple procedure	• Acknowledge distressing emotions, including anger from patient/family as they cope with poor prognosis. • Refocus patient on realistic goals such as optimal symptom control.
Visceral Pain	• Consider contributions of pancreatic insufficiency and constipation to distress. • Consider anesthetic approach, such as celiac plexus block if opioids ineffective, or side effects too problematic. • Cf. Chapter 7, Pain.
Preoccupation with fatigue	• Openly address concerns. • Check lab and give blood transfusion if indicated. • Stimulants such as *methylphenidate* (Ritalin®), *modafinil* (Provigil®) or *dextroamphetamine* can be useful for fatigue/anergia that comes from depression, opioids, and some chemotherapy (gemcitabine). • Cf. Chapter 7, Fatigue.
Preoccupation with low weight	• Openly address concerns. • Consider appetite adjuvants such as *megestrol* (Megace®) , *mirtazapine* (Remeron®) if anxious or depressed; also stimulants such as *methylphenidate* (Ritalin®) or *dextroamphetamine* (Dexedrine®). • Work with family not to focus solely on eating. What other topics could they be focusing on? What is this keeping them from discussing? What does weight loss mean?
Fear of dying	• Openly address concerns. • Help patient to live in the moment, reprioritize. • Assist patient to do an end of life review. • Discuss hospice and where patient wants to die (home, hospital, etc). • Assist patient in talking about end of life issues with family. • Help patients identify unfinished business and complete what is important.

Genitourinary Cancer

For all of the Genitourinary (GU) cancers, primary psychosocial issues are:
- coping with physical changes;
- body image; and
- sexual dysfunction.

Evaluation

Table 9.21 Psychosocial Issues with GU Cancers

Prostate (during early phases of diagnosis)	• General worries of a cancer diagnosis • Controversy about the best primary treatments, i.e., radical prostatectomy, radiation therapy, and "watchful waiting." They show no difference in overall survival or quality of life, but differences in specific areas of functioning, i.e., sexual, urinary or bowel functioning. • Multiple second opinions regarding primary therapy sometimes create more confusion and distress. • Relationship that fosters cofidence and trust of urologist reduces uncertainty. • Reactions depend on psychiatric history, social supports available and significant life changes, such as recent widowhood, divorce and dating, impending or recent retirement, loss of spouses or family members (especially to prostate cancer).
Testicular	• Loss of testis - standard diagnostic procedure is to remove affected testis via inguinal orchiectomy; biopsy alone may spread cells. • Tumor marker anxiety may become a problem and produce anxiety while awaiting results, similar to men with prostate cancer. • Concern for recurrence and treatment side effects. • At peak of a young male adult's development leads to heightened risk of depression, anxiety, anticipation of pain, bodily trauma, fertility, and death.
Non-seminomas	• Fear of dying.
Bladder	• Repeat cystoscopies following local therapy that avoids/postpones cystectomy • Sexual and urinary functioning affected in a similar fashion to radical prostatectomy. • A large proportion of men suffer erectile impotence, though the incidence is decreasing with nerve sparing techniques. • Major sexual side effect for women is genital pain, particularly during intercourse.

(continued, next page)

Table 9.21 Psychosocial Issues with GU Cancers (continued)

Renal carcinoma	• Compromised renal function
	• Poor prognosis major cause for distress
	• Coping with pain, shortness of breath, concentration deficits, cognitive problems
	• As the disease progresses, anticipatory bereavement becomes a pertinent challenge.
	• Complicated by disease-free periods when the person is free of disease after surgery but has the knowledge that recurrence is likely.
	• The conflict of maintaining hope while understanding discouraging odds results in anxiety and depression.

Interventions

Table 9.22 Management of Psychosocial Issues with GU Cancers

Issues with Clinical Treatment	*Management*
Prostatectomy	
• Coping with a significant risk of *erectile dysfunction* (ED) estimated to range from 16% to 82% - most feared side effect	• ED medication: *sildenafil* (Viagra®), *tadalafil* (Cialis®) or *vardenafil* (Levitra®)
	• Penile injections with vasodilating agents
• Coping with *urinary incontinence*	• Vacutainers
• *Fear* of urine leaking, of smelling of urine, and of having to use diapers is humiliating to many men, resulting in shunning social contact.	• Penile suppositories
	• Penile implants
	• Identification of etiologies and medical or surgical resolution (pelvic muscle re-education, bladder training, anticholinergic medications, artificial sphincter surgery)
• Significant *anxiety and depression*	• Educate patients and families about the incontinence
	• Give recommendations to alleviate or reduce symptoms.
	• Cf. Chapter 7, Sexual Dysfunction.
Prostate Cancer - Radiation therapy (conventional or brachytherapy with seed implants)	
• Coping with less risk of *erectile dysfunction and urinary problems* early, but dealing with them later	• *Pain* with boney metastasis
	• Support groups
	• Need for protective undergarments.
• Coping with *bowel function problems* such as anorectal pain, diarrhea, rectal ulceration and bleeding	• Older men are often reluctant to take pain medications or dosages adequate to truly help.
	• Cf. Chapter 7, Pain.
• Coping with a *prostate specific antigen (PSA) level* that does not fall to zero	

(continued, next page)

Table 9.22 Management of Psychosocial Issues with GU Cancers (continued)

Issues with Clinical Treatment	Management

Prostate Cancer - Watchful waiting
- No treatment effect to deal with
- *Anxiety* (33%) about "doing nothing" is difficult for many of these largely older men (over age 70).
- PSA anxiety leads to *insomnia and panic* symptoms.

- Education about PSA levels
- Support and acknowledging fears of rising PSA levels
- Anxiolytic medications: Benzodiazepines such as *alprazolam* (Xanax®), 0.125 mg-0.5 mg prn; *lorazepam* (Ativan®), 0.5 mg - 1 mg prn; or *clonazepam* (Klonopin®), 0.25 mg - 1 mg, prn may be used in the days or weeks prior to PSA testing.
- Antidepressants for more generalized anxiety, e.g., *paroxetine* (Paxil®), *sertraline* (Zoloft®), *venlafaxine* (Effexor®), *citalopram* (Celexa®)

Prostate cancer - Hormonal Treatment (Medical castration with hormones vs. orchiectomy) - Gonadotropin releasing hormone (GnRH) agonists such as leuprolide or goserelin are used in conjunction with antiandrogenic agents that reduce the availability of adrenal androgens, such as flutamide or bicalutamide. Also available are estrogens like diethylstilbestrol. Orchiectomy is less often chosen due to body image issues, despite expense of antiandrogenic medications.

- *Erectile dysfunction and decreased libido; Impact on relationships* - reluctance to participate in therapy, particularly if they have never done so previously
- *Spouses suffer significant distress* coping with their husbands' cancer.
- *Fatigue, muscular weakness* and inability to conduct prior activities
- Concerns about *bodily changes* with gynecomastia or orchiectomy (without prosthesis)
- Contending with *hot flashes* - Symptoms are: diaphoresis; drenching sweats with insomnia; feelings of intense heat, and chills.
- Emotional lability, anxiety, depression and irritability
- Loss of usual ability to focus and diminished concentration

- Education and brief psychotherapies: supportive, cognitive-behavioral, and insight-oriented.
- Often men are more amenable to psychotherapy if the spouse or partner is present.
- Realistic goal setting
- Psychotropic medications can be effective. Start low doses and go slowly (cf. Chapter 4).
- Psychostimulants: *methylphenidate* (Ritalin®) or *modafinil* (Provigil®)
- Activating Antidepressants: *fluoxetine* (Prozac®) or *bupropion* (Wellbutrin®)
- Antidepressants: There have been published positive results with *venlafaxine* (Effexor®), *paroxetine* (Paxil®) and *sertraline* (Zoloft®).
- Pulse the hormonal therapy in 6-12 month intervals.
- Decrease caffeine, alcohol, and hot fluid intake.
- *Sex therapy* with a trained therapist can help a man express the feelings engendered by this dysfunction, and also to help a couple learn alternative ways of sharing sexual intimacy. Cf. Chapter 7, Sexual Dysfunction.

(continued, next page)

Table 9.22 Management of Psychosocial Issues with GU Cancers (continued)

Issues with *Clinical Treatment*	*Management*
Prostate cancer - Hormonal Treatment (continued)	
• Note: Men with a *history of depression* are at greater risk of becoming depressed and should be monitored for symptoms such as losing interest in pleasurable and meaningful activities, social withdrawal, frequent passive or active thoughts about dying, constant worry about the future as a sacrifice to living a fuller life in the present.	(see previous page)
• Absent libido	
• Feeling emasculated	

Prostate cancer - Chemotherapy

• Anxiety/fear, fatigue	• Cf. Chapter 6, Anxiety Disorders and Chapter 7, Fatigue.

Testicular cancer - Retroperitoneal lymph node dissection (RPLND)

• Associated with *ejaculatory dysfunction*, though newer nerve sparing procedures may preserve normal ejaculation. Learning to cope with *infertility and atypical retrograde ejaculation* that is frequently caused by *retroperitoneal lymph node dissection, radiation therapy or chemotherapy* (though sexual desire and ability to have erections and orgasms are usually not affected). Antegrade ejaculation may return spontaneously, months or years after surgery.	• Individual and couples therapy help patient/couple:
	  • develop an understanding of problems;
	  • find new ways of coping;
	  • adapt to changed situation;
	  • address infertility and fears about the effects on sexual functioning, especially before a young man has been involved in a long-term sexual relationship; and
	  • role-play different dating scenarios to lessen anxiety.
	• Individual psychotherapy can help a single or divorced man figure out how to think about and deal with dating and talking about sex with a new partner.

(continued, next page)

Table 9.22 Management of Psychosocial Issues with GU Cancers (continued)

Issues with Clinical Treatment *Management*

Testicular - Orchiectomy with or without chemotherapy

- Adjusting to *change in appearance* due to *unilateral orchiectomy*.
- Dealing with the frustration and quality of life compromises of some late complications of *chemotherapy*: compromised renal function from cisplatin nephrotoxicity, Raynaud's phenomenon following combinations of vinblastine and bleomycin, and neuropathy and ototoxicity attributable to cisplatin and vinblastine leave patients with secondary deficits that challenge their daily living.
- *Decreased sexual activity and diminished intensity of orgasm* are common problems.

- Thorough sexual histories should include questions about frequency and intensity of sexual activity, desire, erection, orgasm, and satisfaction.
- Artificial testicular implants
- Identifying and dealing with decreased sexual interest and avoidance
- Cf. Chapter 7, Sexual Dysfunction.

Bladder cancer - Radical cystectomy, with or without other treatments
(in women also includes hysterectomy, oophorectomy and resection of the anterior wall of the vagina)

- Sexual and urinary functioning affected in a similar fashion to radical prostatectomy.
- A large proportion suffers erectile impotence, though the incidence is decreasing with nerve sparing techniques.
- Major sexual side effect for women is *genital pain, particularly during intercourse*.

- Use of vaginal dilators, lubricants, and estrogen creams help women overcome the scarring and premature menopause.
- Cf. Chapter 7, Sexual Dysfunction.

Bladder cancer - Ileal loop diversion with creation of a permanent stoma

- Concerns about *embarrassment* from odor, leakage, and spills:
  - *negatively impact sexual function* in the patient and partner;
  - *impact social and work environments*; and
  - *commonly cause anxiety, depressed mood, and shunning of social interactions*.
- Women usually make a better adjustment to the presence of a stoma than do men.

- Helped by internal development of urinary reservoirs constructed from bowel. These can be anastomosed to either the skin or urethra. When attached to the urethra, continence can be maintained. This has permitted the creation of the neobladder, with which almost all patients achieve daytime urinary continence.
- Complications are higher than with the conduit. These procedures obviate need for appliance.

(continued, next page)

Table 9.22 Management of Psychosocial Issues with GU Cancers (continued)

Issues with Clinical Treatment	*Management*
Bladder cancer- Preoperative chemotherapy with or without radiation sometimes used before cystectomy	
• *Fear* of possible cystectomy after long periods of treatments to save bladder. • *Anxiety* at unknown future.	• Address fear and anxiety. • Medicate, if indicated. • Cf. Chapter 4; Chapter 6, Anxiety Disorders.
Renal carcinoma - Radical nephrectomy for localized disease	
• Complicated by disease-free periods when the person is free of disease after surgery but has the knowledge that recurrence is likely. • The conflict of maintaining hope while understanding discouraging odds results in *anxiety and depression*.	• Cf. Chapter 6, Anxiety Disorders and Mood Disorders.
Renal carcinoma - Preservation with only partial excision of renal tissue	
• Anxiety	• Maintain realistic hope.
Renal carcinoma - Chemotherapy	
• Depression, anxiety, cognitive dysfunction and delirium.	• Support and medication for anxiety or depressive symptoms, with consideration of renal functioning • Cf. Chapter 6, Anxiety Disorders, Mood Disorders and Cognitive Disorders.
Renal carcinoma - Immunotherapy, autolymphocyte therapy, vaccines and nonspecific immunomodulators: Interferon-alpha and interleukin-2 (IL-2)	
(Interferon-alpha and IL-2 have been used with some success in treating advanced renal cancer.) • The first two may be mediated through physical or somatic side effects (e.g., fatigue, fever). • Depression, anxiety, cognitive dysfunction and delirium	• Prophylactic use of *SSRI antidepressants* such as *paroxetine* (Paxil®) decreases fatigue and depression. • Cf. Chapter 4; Chapter 6, Anxiety Disorders, Mood Disorders and Cognitive Disorders; Chapter 7, Fatigue.

Summary

Most prominent psychosocial issues in GU tumors are coping with changes in sexuality, bladder and bowel function, body image, relationships, and lifestyle. In prostate cancer, libido is directly affected by hormonal treatments, whereas in the other GU cancers, it is physical sexual functioning that is primarily affected. In both prostate and testicular cancers, tumor markers that are used to follow treatment outcomes create significant anxiety. In bladder and renal cell tumors, guilt for having been a smoker complicates reaction to illness. Urinary incontinence is a common, transient problem with any of the GU cancers, however it is a longer term problem for those with prostate and bladder cancers. Patients with either prostate or renal cell cancers must deal with the pain of bone metastases in advanced disease, and knowledge of poor prognosis.

Management of these problems is best done by means of:
- education and Support about illness and treatment;
- individual and Group Psychotherapy;
- couples therapy;
- behavioral and Relaxation Interventions;
- psychotropic medications for symptoms of distress; and
- referral to a specialist for erectile dysfunction or to a sex counselor.

Gynecological Cancer

Introduction

The gynecological cancers present a special set of psychosocial problems, which are common to all: ovary, uterus, cervix, vagina and vulva. The problems vary by site, but all women experience a common set of emotional difficulties. Screening is imperfect and not universally used, so diagnosis is sometimes missed and/or delayed. Because gynecological cancer is less common than breast cancer, support from others is less readily available; and it is common to have a great sense of guilt, feelings of being alone and poorly understood. The most common problems and recommended approach are listed below.

Table 9.23 Gynecological Cancer - Common Problems and Approaches[43]

Stigma and embarrassment	Steady support; clear commitment to patient's care and well-being
Fears of disability and death	Clear explanations/options
Threat to sexuality, intimacy, fertility, and elimination	Convey sense of being competent and compassionate. Openly address these issues instead of waiting for the patient to bring it up.
Loneliness, fear, anger, grief	Referral to social supports in community; when distress is high: Offer support, information, and medications as needed.
Loss of control; Difficulty for caregiver to ask for help	Give patient options, accurate information.

There are **inaccurate or painful associations** of gynecological cancer that contribute to the patient's sense of guilt, fear and isolation.

Table 9.24 Myths about Gynecological Cancer

Ovarian	Causes early death
Cervical	Caused by patient's promiscuity or irresponsibility
Fallopian, vaginal, vulvar	Greater feeling of isolation, because these types of cancer are rare

Evaluation

Include a psychiatric assessment as part of the initial work-up so that special attention to patient's distress may prevent major psychological barriers to treatment adherence.

Table 9.25 Initial Workup - Questions for a Quick Psychiatric Assessment

Psychiatry history	Prior substance abuse? Prior psychiatric treatment? Prior suicide attempt? Family psychiatric treatment?
Social history	Present social support: family, friends, church. Is stable support present?
Present coping	Is patient largely dealing realistically with the diagnosis? Treatment plans? Currently using psychotropic medications? Who, what, where, when, and how?
Level of distress (cf. Chapter 2)	Distress Thermometer: "On a scale of 0-10, how distressed are you?" For score of 5 or greater, algorithm indicates referral to mental health or social resources, depending on the cause of distress. Problem list: what are the carriers for distress?

Interventions

Interventions which can be initiated by the oncologist are outlined on the following pages in Table 9.26. Guidelines for determining when to refer a patient for psychiatric evaluation or treatment are listed in Table 9.27.

Table 9.26 Gynecological Cancer - Interventions[43 - 48]

Problem and Causes	*Interventions*

Anxiety (cf. Chapter 6, Anxiety) peaks as treatment starts, falls during treatment, then peaks again as it ends

Problem and Causes	Interventions
• Fear of illness/death	• Reassurance by team

• Preexisting psychiatric disorder (anxiety, panic, phobias, obsessive compulsive)
• Withdrawal states
• Pulmonary embolus
	• Medicate appropriately:*
	  • Benzodiazepine: *lorazepam* (Ativan®); *clonazepam* (Klonopin®) ; *alprazolam* (Xanax®)
	  • For preexisting or chronic anxiety disorders, add SSRI: *fluoxetine* (Prozac®); *escitalopram* (Lexapro) *sertraline* (Zoloft®)
	  • Antipsychotics: *olanzapine* (Zyprexa®); *risperidone* (Risperdol®)
	  • Insomnia: *eszopiclone* (Lunesta®); *zolpidem* (Ambien®); *zolpidem SR* (Ambien CR); *temazepam* (Restoril®); *trazodone* (Desyrel®)
	• Behavioral techniques for insomnia

• Medication side effects	• If anxiety is due to restless legs from phenothiazine or atypical antipsychotic side effects: *diphenhydramine* (Benadryl®) ; *benztropine* (Cogentin®)
• Hypoxia	• Oxygen
• Fear of recurrence	• Continued monitoring
• Pain, uncontrolled; metabolic disorders	• Manage pain, other physical side effects. • Refer to mental health professional if symptoms persist

Depression (cf. Chapter 6, Mood Disorders)

Problem and Causes	Interventions
• Response to loss of fertility (grief)	• Acknowledge grief; refer to grief counselor or support group. Commitment to continuing care is crucial to coping.
• Changed appearance/role	• Rule out medication causes (steroids); manage pain and other physical side effects.

(continued, next page)

* Cf. Chapter 4.

Table 9.26 Gynecological Cancer - Interventions (continued)[43 - 48]

Problem and Causes	Interventions

Depression (continued) (cf. Chapter 6, Mood Disorders)

- Note: symptoms of depression mimic illness-related decreased libido, anorexia, fatigue, insomnia
  - Consider medications:*
    - SSRI: *escitalopram* (Lexapro®); *fluoxetine* (Prozac®); *sertraline* (Zoloft®); *citalopram* (Celexa®); *paroxetine* (Paxil®)
    - SNRI: *venlafaxine* (Effexor®); *duloxetine* (Cymbalta®)
    - Others: *bupropion* (Wellbutrin®); *mirtazapine* (Remeron®)
  - If fatigue is significant, psychostimulant: *methylphenidate* (Ritalin®); *modafinil* (Provigil®)

- Sexual dysfunction
  - Refer to sexual rehabilitation program, or to marital or psychiatric therapy.
  - Cf. Chapter 7, Sexual Dysfunction.

Sexual Dysfunction- Libido, arousal-vaginal dryness, dyspareunia, orgasm, relationship issues (cf. Chapter 7, Sexual Dysfunction)

- Side effect of chemotherapies (neuropathy also affects clitoris)
  - Acknowledge sexual changes instead of waiting for the patient to address it.

- Decreased libido
- Relationship issues
- Change in appearance ("damaged goods")
  - Refer to sexual rehabilitation program, or to marital or psychiatric therapy.

- Alteration in hormone production
  - Information, respect, and support regarding hormone replacement (risks and benefits- cancer/ cardiac/cognition/bone)
  - Complementary/ integrative supplements: Soy; Black cohosh; L-arginine; Wild Yam cream

- Shortened vagina
- Vaginal stenosis from radiation
  - Give vaginal dilators 6 weeks after radiation finished.
  - Vaginal water-soluble lubricants: Astroglide®; K-Y Jelly/Liquid®
  - Vaginal moisturizers: Replens®; Vagifem®
  - Sensate focus exercises

- Change in vulvar sensation postoperative
  - Erotic devices

*Cf. Chapter 4.

(continued, next page)

Table 9.26 Gynecological Cancer - Interventions (continued)[43 - 48]

Problem and Causes	Interventions
Premature Menopause	
• Hot flashes	• *Venlafaxine* (EffexorXR®) • SSRIs also help with symptoms: *fluoxetine* (Prozac®) ; *paroxetine* (Paxil®)* • Other: *clonidine* (Catapres®); *neurontin* (Gabapentin®); Vitamin E; Ginseng; Black cohosh; Wild yam; Soy isoflavones • Diet: control weight; no caffeine, spicy foods or alcohol • Dress in layers.
• Vaginal dryness • Vaginal atrophy • Vulvar atrophy	• Vaginal moisturizers and lubricants • Estring® vaginally; estrogen vaginal cream • Soy
• Mood instability	• SSRI: *fluoxetine* (Prozac®); *sertraline* (Zoloft®) ; *citalopram* (Celexa®); *escitalopram* (Lexapro®)*
• Insomnia	• Medicate prn: *lorazepam* (Ativan®); *zolpidem* (Ambien®) ; *temazepam* (Restoril®); *eszopiclone* (Lunesta®); *trazodone* (Desryl®)
• Migraine headaches	• Rule out metastasis, then treat pain.
• Body aroma change • Skin and hair changes	• Body creams and lotions
Infertility	
• Depression, grief	• Treat depression. • Refer to group.
• Loss of choice	• Surrogacy, adoption • Preservation of fertility when possible
• Fear of continuing/new relationship (great risk for relationship less than 5 yrs)	• Refer for marital or individual therapy; group therapy.

*Cf. Chapter 4.

(continued, next page)

Table 9.26 Gynecological Cancer - Interventions (continued)[43-48]

Problem and Causes	*Interventions*
Survivorship	
• Delayed reactions	• Continued monitoring
• Fear of recurrence (late recurrence, 5-10 years, always a threat)	• Reassurance

• Slow progression creates profound, intense therapeutic situation:
  • Early recurrences - cancer as chronic disease
  • Later recurrences - quality *vs.* duration of life
	• Change treatment options.
	• Comfort care
	• Address communication issues.

• Preparing for dying and death	• Coordination with hospice, nursing staff
• Hypervigilance • Family/friends	• Support groups
• Dating issues, e.g., when/how to tell new partner?	• Support groups
• Sexual dysfunction • Body image	• Refer for sexual counseling/psychiatric intervention.
• Medical sequelae of treatment • Neuropathy	• Neuropathies: *neurontin* (Gabapentin®); *amitriptyline* (Elavil®); *duloxetine* (Cymbalta®); *venlafaxine* (EffexorXR®)*
• Cardiac	• Monitor.
• Bowel (long-term effect of radiation)	• Treat diarrhea/constipation with medication, diet.
• Bladder (Incontinence, urgency, increased UTIs)	• Kegel exercises • No caffeine

(continued, next page)   *Cf. Chapter 4.

Table 9.26 Gynecological Cancer - Interventions (continued)[43-48]

Problem and Causes	Interventions
Survivorship (continued)	
• Bone	• Bone density at baseline and annually
	• **Medicate:** alendronate (Fosamax) weekly or daily; pamidronate (Aredia) IV monthly; zoledronic acid (Zometa) IV monthly
	• Calcium + Vit. D- 1000mg/d; calcitonin Nasal spray daily
	• Tobacco avoidance
	• Daily weight-bearing exercise
• Cognitive	• Neuro- cognitive testing before and after treatment

Table 9.27 When to refer patients for psychiatric evaluation or treatment

- Patients experiencing **intense or overwhelming anxiety** or any other symptoms of:

Major denial	Dissociation
Psychosis	Delirium (disorientation, confusion, memory problems)

- Patients with **previous history or family history of:**

Depression	Suicide attempt
Substance abuse	Psychiatric hospitalization

- Patients who during cancer treatment require **maintenance of:**

Psychotropic medications	Steroids

- Patients displaying **hostile or inappropriate behavior towards family or staff**

- Patients experiencing **difficulty making treatment decisions or complying with treatment**

- Patients dealing with other **concomitant life stressors**

- Patients who have **special issues** with regard to:

Age	Fertility
Support	Beliefs
Previous experience with cancer	Previous experience with death in the family

- Patients considering **higher-risk decisions about fertility preservation versus cancer treatment**

- Patients considering **end-of-active treatment decisions**

Head and Neck Cancer

Table 9.28 Treatment Strategies for Nicotine and Alcohol Withdrawal

Smoking Cessation	Treatment Strategies
Nicotine withdrawal - 85% of head and neck cancers are associated with prior tobacco use.	Pharmacotherapy Anti-craving medication • *bupropion* (Wellbutrin SR®) 150mg/day for 3 days, then 150mg bid for 3 months Benzodiazepines for anxiety • *lorazepam* (Ativan®) 0.5mg - 1.0mg bid (12-hour half-life) • *clonazepam* (Klonopin®) 0.25mg - 1.0mg at bedtime (24-hour half-life) • *alprazolam* (Xanax®) 0.25mg - 0.5mg bid Nicotine replacement therapy - Do not use nicotine replacement if plastic surgery involves free flap as vasoconstriction may damage graft: • Dosage for Patch (Nicoderm CQ®, Prostep®, Nicotrol®): • If smoking 11 cig/24hr or less: give 21mg/24hr (6 weeks); then 14mg/24hr (2 weeks); then 7mg/24hrs (2 weeks) • If smoking 10 cig/24hr or more: give 14mg/24hrs (6 weeks); then 7mg/24hrs (2 weeks) *or* with Nicotrol® -15mg/16hrs (6 weeks); 10mg/16hrs (2 weeks); 5mg/16hrs (2 weeks) • Dosage for Inhaler (Nicotrol® Inhaler — buccal absorption from puffs) 6 to 16 cartridges per 24 hr period — several inhalations over 20 minutes (Up to 6 months)
Continued smoking increases rates of recurrence and second primary cancers.	Motivational counseling • Identify stage: pre-contemplative, contemplative, ready • Promote increase in motivation with education regarding risks
Up to 33% continue or relapse with tobacco use.	Behavioral counseling • Identify cues, social circumstances, triggers to reduce smoking. • Explore avoidance.

(continued, next page)

Table 9.28 Treatment Strategies for Nicotine and Alcohol Withdrawal (continued)

Risk factors for continued smoking include less severe disease (e.g. mouth compared to larynx) and less extensive treatment, younger age and heavy smokers (greater dependence) .

Cognitive therapy
* Evaluate self-esteem, self beliefs.
* Affirm strengths while countering negative attitudes.

Alcohol Withdrawal
One standard drink contains 10g of alcohol (285cc of full-strength beer, 100cc of wine or 30cc of spirits). Withdrawal symptoms usually appear within 6 to 24 hours of the last consumption of alcohol and typically persist for 72 hours, but may last longer. Best practice: identify high risk patients ahead of admission and plan a prophylactic regimen of medication to suppress or modify withdrawal symptoms in vulnerable patients.

Treatment Strategies
Potential prophylaxis regimens include:
* shorter acting benzodiazepine if there is concern about liver function or respiratory function, e.g., *lorazepam* (Ativan®) 2 mg q 6h for 4 doses, then 1 mg q 6 h for 8 doses
* longer acting benzodiazepine if there is no concern about liver function or respiratory function, e.g., *diazepam* (Valium®) 10 mg q 6 h for 4 doses, then 5 mg q 6 h for 8 doses

Add Thiamine and B group vitamins.

Acute withdrawal symptoms: tremor, sweats, anxiety, agitation, nausea and vomiting

Symptomatic management:
* Shorter-acting benzodiazepines if concern about liver function or respiratory function: *lorazepam* (Ativan®) challenge — 2 mg hourly until patient becomes settled, sleepy but arousable. Take the total dose needed to achieve a sleepy state and divide into a 6 hourly regimen for the next day. Taper over 3 subsequent days.
* Give intravenous fluids, thiamine, folate, and multivitamins as indicated.

Severe withdrawal symptoms: perceptual disturbances and seizures; delirium tremens, wherein disorientation, confusion and hallucinations also emerge

Longer-acting benzodiazepine if there is no concern about liver function or respiratory function: *diazepam* (Valium®) 10 - 20 mg, 1 - 2 hourly until symptoms subside and a sleepy state is induced. A cumulative dose of 60 mg usually is sufficient. Taper over 3 subsequent days. If agitation and hallucinations emerge, add *haloperidol* (Haldol®) 0.5 - 2 mg tid to qid. Consider a *gabapentin* (Neurontin®) regimen if there is considerable concern about liver function.

Medical emergency: fever, tachycardia and dehydration

Emergency medical treatment

Table 9.29 Difficult Symptoms for Distressed Head and Neck Cancer Patients

Symptom/Problem	Treatment
Xerostomia - lack/thickening of saliva, especially after radiotherapy (affects speech, mastication and swallowing)	• Prophylactic amifostine during radiation treatment may reduce • Dry mouth can be relieved by artificial sialogogues; frequent drinks; and *pilocarpine* (Salagen®) 2.5, 5.0, 10 mg, tid to stimulate saliva (side effect: sweating).
Trouble swallowing psychotropic medications	The following medications are sublinqual or swallowed more easily: • For depression: *mirtazepine* (Remeron®) sol tabs, *sertraline* (Zoloft®) liquid, *paroxetine* (Paxil®) liquid • For anxiety: *clonazepam* (Klonopin®) Wafers • For restlessness: *olanzapine* (Zyprexa®, Zydis®), *risperidone* (Risperdal®) M-tabs
Local mouth pain	• Equal parts of 2% viscous *lidocaine* (Xylocaine®), *diphenhydramine* (Benadryl®) and *aluminum hydroxide – magnesium hydroxide* (Mylanta®) — 10 ml of mouth wash/gargle for 60 seconds pre-meals, and bedtime q 3 h • *benzocaine* (Orajel®) ointment on tongue
Nutrition problems	• Consider Percutaneous Endoscopic Gastrostomy (PEG) versus nasogastric feeding. • Use food diary, supplements, nutritionist; maintain presurgical weight. • Dumping Syndrome: decrease fluid with frequent small meals.
Dysphagia	• Refer to speech pathologist for swallowing rehabilitation.
Tracheostomy	• Change from cuffed to uncuffed 5-7 days post surgery. • Suctioning every 2 hours; clean inner canula every 4 hours. • Aerosol bronchodilator (eg. albuterol)
Intraoral obturators and dental prosthetics	• Obturator plates close defects; irrigate with mixture of 1 quart water, 1 teaspoon baking soda and 1 teaspoon salt.
Mucositis	• Water and salt rinses; *sucralfate* (Carafate®) oral suspension • benzydamine 0.15% solution, rinse q 3-6 h
Skin Care	• hydrophilic gels (aloe vera) tid; sunscreens longterm • Long-term dry desquamation: add 0.5% hydrocortisone cream. • Moist desquamation: silver *sulfadiazine* (Silvadene®) ointment; nonstick dressings

Table 9.30 Treatments for Psychosocial Issues with Head and Neck Cancer

Disfigurement and body image	• Sensitivity to shame and stigma • Sit with patient and mirror to discuss appearance when dressings have been taken down. • Promote control, shared decision-making, and openness to wear prosthesis .
Distress and depression >40%[49]	• Check for depressive symptoms and social withdrawal. • Explore role of family and friends, partner. • Ask about sexual functioning as a marker for adaptive rehabilitation. • Check for demoralization or loss of meaning.
Speech rehabilitation - Post-total laryngectomy: 52% report hyposmia (less ability to smell); 15% report dysgeusia (trouble with taste); and 38% report nasal discharge.[50]	Options: • Speech therapy to gain esophageal speech (20 - 30%) • Use of electropharynx (40 - 55%) • Tracheoesophageal punctures, cricopharyngeal myotomies
Patient attitudes about goals and quality of life[51]	• Cure: 75% of patients rank first; 93% rank in top 3 • Long life: 56% rank in top 3 • Free of pain: 35% rank in top 3 • Normal energy and activities: 24% rank in top 3 • Swallowing, speech, appearance, chewing: 10 - 20% rank in top 3
Active treatment of advanced head and neck cancer[52] - 30% report swallowing, hoarseness and mouth pain at 12 months, xerostomia, loss of taste	• Need for soft diet is prominent.
Advanced disease of the head and neck[53,54] - associated with trismus, xerostomia, sticky saliva	• Social withdrawal and stigma, swallowing and speech problems
Quality of Life measures	• University of Washington QoL Instrument[55] • EORTC Head and Neck Module[54] • FACT Head and Neck Module[56]

Hematological Cancer

The diagnosis of any hematological malignancy results in fear and pessimism due to the wide perception that diseases of the blood are serious and often fatal. Treatment decisions must sometimes be made quickly before the patient and family can process the emotional impact of the diagnosis. Others must deal with "watchful waiting" despite hearing what they perceive as a dire diagnosis. Patients consent for intensive treatment with the hope of achieving remission or cure while at the same time fearing death, discomfort, dependence on others, and coping with disruptions in their lives. Chronic forms of these malignancies often have many treatment options. The prolonged course makes patient's realization of a terminal phase difficult.

Table 9.31 Psychosocial Problems Common to all Hematological Malignancies

- Diseases of the "blood stream" and lymph nodes are highly feared by the public.
- Disease that is systemic and not localized to any single part of the body; it cannot be "cut out" like solid tumors
- Fears of disability and death
- Uncertainty of future for self and family
- Disrupted life plans/ education/ career or job/ retirement
- Fear of pain
- Loss of control and helpless feelings
- Fatigue and diminished energy; anemia is often chronic and debilitating
- Fear of blood transfusions

Table 9.32 Overriding Psychosocial Problems with Hematological Malignancies

- Impact on fertility; risk that disease or treatment may injure future offspring
- Impact on sexuality; premature menopause and decreased libido
- Post-traumatic distress disorder symptoms after all intensive therapies
- Financial concerns, especially for breadwinner
- Isolation and separation from others with aggressive therapies to decrease infections
- Fears of "chemo brain," cognitive impairment from treatment or illness
- Changes in appearance and body image

Table 9.33 Treatments for Psychological/ Psychosocial Problems Associated with Distinct Hematological Malignancies

Acute Lymphoblastic Leukemia (ALL)

- Peaks in adults around 50 - 60 years of age
- Dealing with side effects of induction therapy (vincristine, prednisone, and anthracycline) and consolidation
- CNS treatment and prophylaxisIntrathecal methotrexate continues throughout induction/ consolidation/ maintenance with single or combination agents including methotrexate/cytarabine/steroids/ radiation
- Consideration of allogeneic stem cell transplant (SCT) for high risk patients; debate about prognostic factors of allogeneic bone marrow transplant (BMT)
- Maintenance treatment for two years of combination chemotherapy
- Allogeneic stem cell transplant for patients in second remission, phase I and II trials of new agents for treatment resistant ALL when potentially curative allogeneic BMT is not possible

- Support for patient and caregiver through intensive multi-chemotherapy; induction, consolidation (with CNS prophylaxis) and intensification, and maintenance
- Help with facing treatment toxicity and mortality.
- Monitor mood, fatigue, neuropathy, constipation, infections, disseminated intravascular coagulation (DIC), compliance with frequent hospitalizations, clinic visits, and white cell growth factors at home. (Cf. Chapters 6, 7.)
- Treat with anti-depressant and anti- anxiety agents. Psychostimulants for fatigue; Steroid-related mood and sleep disorders treated with mood- stabilizing neuroleptics. (Cf. Chapter 6, Anxiety, Mood Disorders.)
- Monitor mood states and cognitive deficits (concentration, memory, confusion). (Cf. Chapter 6, Cognitive Disorders.)
- Adequate information about benefits and risks versus continued chemotherapy to make informed decisions
- Family/ donor issues for allogeneic SCT
- Coping with uncertainty of future
- Coping with relapse, which is common; symptoms of fatigue, cognitive deficits
- Dealing with uncertainty; commitment to long- term treatment and prolonged disruption of life tasks
- Disappointment of relapse and dealing with fears of finding a donor for transplant and its many unknowns
- Awareness of protocols in ALL- maintains hope in the face of poor prognosis

Acute Myeloid Leukemia (AML)

- Largely after 40, median around 60.
- Induction more intensive, and relapses are often earlier than for ALL. Prognostic groups better defined for AML.
- Awareness of high relapse rate; higher treatment morbidity/ mortality over 60

- Adaptation to diagnosis of AML often in context of bruising, bleeding, fatigue, fever, transfusions, DIC, and low platelet counts
- Emotional support for patient and caregiver
- Treat fatigue, depression, anxiety, insomnia, anorexia, and pain. (Cf. Chapters 6, 7.)
- Help with risk- benefit analysis to facilitate decision making about investigational protocols (quality vs. quantity of life), supportive symptom control, existential concerns for patient and caregiver; anticipatory grief-referral for support.

(continued, next page)

Table 9.33   Treatments for Psychological/ Psychosocial Problems Associated with Distinct Hematological Malignancies (continued)

Acute Myeloid Leukemia (AML) (continued)

- Treatment is generally consolidated into less than one year; usually includes cytarabine and antracycline.
- Consideration of transplant options; mini- transplants now an option for older patients.
- Multiply relapsed AML and not a candidate for transplantation: Investigational protocols.

(see previous page)

Chronic Lymphocytic Leukemia (CLL)

- Most common adult leukemia; often asymptomatic in older adults (median age 65); no treatment until symptomatic from the disease
- *Advanced stage:* Investigational protocols; new therapies available offer reason for hope despite advancing disease.

- Support for patients who are unable to tolerate "watchful waiting" without treatment
- Anxiety about clinical progression with symptoms of night sweats, weight loss, anorexia, and infections
- Supportive symptom control: Fatigue (psycho-stimulant), insomnia (hypnotics), depression, anxiety (antidepressants and anxiolytics), pain control, demoralization common with decreased ability to function and to enjoy activities; erythropoietic growth factor important to control fatigue. (Cf. Chapters 6, 7.)

Chronic Myelocytic Leukemia (CML)

- *Chronic Phase:* More common in older adults (median age 60's); Treatment with *imatinib* (Gleevec®)
- Hydroxyurea maybe used transiently with Gleevec®; new investigational agents designed for Gleevec® resistance
- Consideration of SCT for younger patients with early failure and HLA-matched sibling donor

(continued, next page)

- Control drug side effects (muscle cramps, rash, GI upset, weight gain, edema) with supportive measures.
- Patients often have significant worries about what happens when/if Gleevec® doesn't work.
- Emphasize compliance with medication even when patients 'feel normal'.
- Assist patient and family to assess benefits (possibly curative) against risks of SCT to facilitate decision making about the transplant.
- Treat symptoms related to chemotherapy — fatigue, fevers, etc. (Cf. Chapter 7, Fatigue.)
- Increased awareness/ need for counseling related to existential concerns
- Help sustain hope by providing information about trials.

Table 9.33 Treatments for Psychological/ Psychosocial Problems Associated with Distinct Hematological Malignancies (continued)

Chronic Myelocytic Leukemia (CML) (continued)

- *Accelerated Phase:* Higher dose *imatinib* (Gleevec®); chronic phase and Phase II studies in trial for Gleevec resistance. Realization of need for SCT. Possible intensive chemotherapy (cytarabine/ anthracycline or vincristine/ prednisone) prior SCT to regain chronic phase.
- *Blastic Phase:* Responses are short; consideration of transplant but with limited expectations of benefit. Need for chemotherapy similar to 'accelerated phase' to try to achieve remission. High rates of failure with any therapy.

- High dose Gleevec® has greater effect on quality of life.
- Treat symptoms related to chemotherapy.
- Counseling for anticipated grief; support for caregiver/ family.

Hodgkin's Disease

- Occurs at younger adult age (third decade peak), and after 45; associated with good prognosis and high cure rate
- *Limited Early Disease:* Radiation therapy alone
- *Intermediate or advanced disease:* ABVD, or alternating with MOPP; and combined modality with radiation (ABVD is adriamycin, bleomycin, vinblastine, dacarbazine; MOPP is mechlorethamine, vincristine, prednisone, procarbazine.)
- *Recurrent Disease:* High dose chemotherapy with autologous SCT
- *Long Term Sequelae:* Cardiac, fertility, secondary malignancies, hypothyroidism

- Patients have fewer fears of death, but focus on treatment side effects (short and long term).
- Fear of future for children and family
- Symptom control measures: fatigue (psycho-stimulant), anxiety, depression, insomnia, nausea, esophageal symptoms. (Cf. Chapters 6, 7.)
- Treat immediate symptoms of therapy-fatigue, nausea, neuropathy, constipation. (Cf. Chapter 7.)
- Help in coping with infections, hospitalizations and especially in young patients with change in body image. Treatment given as outpatient is very disruptive to normal life.
- Assist patients and families with concerns about less intensive therapy and risk of relapse vs. more intensive therapy early and its potential long-term effects such as sterility and late secondary malignancies.
- Reassurance of potential cure
- Assist patients and family in dealing with hospitalizations and long confinement, disruption of routine life, and some uncertainty of cure.

(continued, next page)

Table 9.33 Treatments for Psychological/ Psychosocial Problems Associated with Distinct Hematological Malignancies (continued)

Hodgkin's Disease (continued)

- Evaluate psychosocial factors prior to transplant; monitor symptoms during SCT.
- Monitor for signs of delirium secondary to opioids/ infection- treat with neuroleptics.
- Optimize pain control; fatigue management options.
- Some combination regimens cause sterility; sperm-banking for men, adequate information for women (counseling regarding fertility options), sexual dysfunction.
- Monitor thyroid and other endocrine abnormalities and related mood disorders.
- Monitor treatment-related post-traumatic stress disorder symptoms.

Non- Hodgkin's Lymphoma

• Most common in older adults and men.	• Information about type of lymphoma and treatment options
• *Indolent Lymphomas:* May be curable or quite indolent	• Emphasize appropriate early treatment for improved outcome in many early stage lymphomas.
• MALT Lymphomas — may be associated with certain infections and autoimmune disease. Often localized at diagnosis; surgery or radiation therapy; may be curable at early stage. Alkylating agents and fludarabine used systemically for more advanced disease.	• Treatment of associated diseases • Adapt to side effects of local surgery and radiation. • Assist patient in being informed about appropriate therapy, adjusting to diagnosis, and pursuing treatment quickly. • Help adapt to "watchful waiting" without treatment for advanced stage.
• Low Grade Follicular — early stage may be curable with radiation	• Treat when symptoms develop. • Assure that patient understands options.
• *Advance stage indolent lymphomas*: Single agent and combination chemotherapy; involved field radiations, monoclonal antibodies; autologous or allogeneic SCT; may transform to diffuse large cell	• Information about treatment options • Supportive symptom control (fatigue, pain, insomnia, neuropathy) from disease and therapy • Monitor for development of depression and anxiety. • Risk of graft vs. host disease with physical and psychological sequelae following allogeneic transplant • Symptom control (pain, fatigue, insomnia, cardiac toxicity, alopecia), demoralization related to aggressive treatment
(continued, next page)	• Hematopoietic growth factors to reduce toxicity of treatment

Table 9.33 Treatments for Psychological/ Psychosocial Problems Associated with Distinct Hematological Malignancies (continued)

Non- Hodgkin's Lymphoma (continued)

- *Aggressive Lymphomas*: Diffuse Large B-Cell; CHOP (cyclophosphamide, doxorubicin, vincristine, prednisone) and rituximab, other combination chemotherapy and autologous/ allogeneic SCT; potentially curable. Treatment is initiated early with combination chemotherapy and SCT.
- Mantle Cell: Combination chemotherapies and monoclonal antibody (CHOP and rituximab) or hyper CVAD +/- autologous transplant; aggressive form not curable
- For aggressive lymphomas: increasing use of FDA approved monoclonal antibodies: rituximab, ^{90}Y- ibritumumab, ^{131}I- tositumomab, Alemtuzumab.

- Symptom control (pain, fatigue, insomnia, cardiac toxicity, alopecia), demoralization related to aggressive treatment. (Cf. Chapters 6, 7.)
- Counseling for distress related to poor prognosis; existential concerns; symptom control; monitor for steroid- related mood disorders
- Better tolerated regimens and better quality of life during treatment, but uncertainty about outcome and duration of response

High Grade Lymphomas

- Burkitt's lymphoma and lymphoblastic lymphoma are potentially curable with intensive chemotherapy. Allogeneic transplant for patients with poor prognostic features. Need for CNS prophylaxis in some patients

- Monitor coping with treatment side effects.

Multiple Myeloma

- Occurs in older men and women (median age is in 60s).
- *Early disease:* Asymptomatic "watchful waiting"

- Monitor adaptation to a disease known not to be curable.
- Managing anxiety related to not being in active treatment.
- Monitor for development of depression and anxiety, treat with anti- anxiety/ anti depressant agents.

(continued, next page)

Table 9.33 Treatments for Psychological/ Psychosocial Problems Associated with Distinct Hematological Malignancies (continued)

Multiple Myeloma (continued)

- *Symptomatic disease:* Pain, fractures, anemia, infections; treatment with melphalan +/- prednisone, high dose VAD (vincristine, adriamycin, dexamethasone), high dose steroids, and autologous SCT
- *Relapsed myeloma:* Newer therapies approved by the FDA Thalidomide and bortezomib (Velcade) with dexamethasone; autologous or mini allogeneic SCT in younger patients — still investigational

- Coping with chronic illness with uncomfortable physical symptoms: bone pain/ fragility/ fractures (optimize pain control), infections (prophylaxis-antibiotics and immunoglobulin), neutropenia (G-CSF)
- Monitor for signs of demoralization /depression (antidepressant); mood/ cognitive changes related to hypercalcemia, opioids and steroids; fatigue (psychostimulant). (Cf. Chapters 6, 7.)
- Counseling to find meaning despite chronic illness.
- Optimize symptom control (pain, fatigue, insomnia, peripheral neuropathy). (Cf. Chapter 7.)
- Monitor for steroid- related changes in mood and cognition.
- Drug related effects: thalidomide - asthenia, neuropathy, constipation, headache
- Bortezomib effects: edema, mood change, pain, GI changes, anorexia

Hematopoietic Stem Cell Transplant (HSCT)

Hematopoietic stem cell transplant (HSCT) is an aggressive treatment used for several hematologic malignancies: leukemia, lymphoma, myelodysplastic syndrome, aplastic anemia, and multiple myeloma often after the failure of other treatments. HSCT patients face physical and psychological stressors of hospitalization with physical and social isolation for weeks to months. Treatment away from home and family and friends in cancer centers is difficult. Coping with painful side effects or mucositis, fatigue, isolation and infections complicates coping. Increased dependence on others, long periods of enhanced susceptibility to infections and stress on caregivers during hospitalization and the first 100 days after transplant.

Table 9.34 Psychiatric Pre-Transplant Evaluation

General Considerations

- Adequate understanding of procedure
- Ability to collaborate with the team in long- term care relationships
- Ability to maintain compliance with treatment and make long- term life- style changes
- Availability and quality of social support
- Psychiatric comorbidity

(continued, next page)

Table 9.34 Psychiatric Pre-Transplant Evaluation (continued)

Specific Evaluation	Patient's Primary Caregiver
• Psychiatric history	• Quality of relationship
• Substance abuse history	• Availability of support for primary caregiver
• Psychosocial history	• Other responsibilities (in addition to caring for patient)
• History of trauma	
• Prior history of coping	• Understanding of patient's illness and treatment
• Coping with illness and treatment	
• Compliance with past treatments	• Other current stressors
• Health behaviors	• Health and emotional concerns
• Understanding of illness and treatment (appropriate to education level)	• Coping styles
• Mental status, current psychiatric symptoms	
• Ethnic, cultural, spiritual considerations that may affect treatment	
• Other current stressors	

Given the length and intensity of treatment, it is important to have a thorough pre-transplant psychosocial evaluation to identify those at risk for development of psychosocial morbidity and to initiate early interventions to optimize adaptation to illness and treatment. During hospitalization, patients cope with prolonged periods of isolation with restrictions on visitors and mobility, side effects of chemotherapy and radiation, diminished stamina and cognitive activity. Oral mucositis is the most distressing side effect of myeloablative regimens, and necessitates use of analgesics and reliance on total parenteral nutrition. New agents such as palifermin (Kepivance) are reducing the side effects of therapy such as mucositis. Opioid analgesics used to treat mucositis pain may cause visual hallucinations, confusion, disorientation, vivid frightening dreams, impaired concentration and memory. Monitoring for confusional states related to opioid use, metabolic, renal, hepatic abnormalities and infection is important during chemotherapy and HSCT.

HSCT patients also experience decline in neurocognitive function with up to 60% of patients manifesting mild to moderate cognitive impairment over two years after the transplant, though most patients who experience generalized cognitive decline at 80 days post transplant recover their pre-transplant level of functioning at 1 year follow up. Educating patients about neurocognitive side effects of treatment such as diminished concentration, short-term memory and decreased speed of information processing, and their temporary nature may reduce anxiety and facilitate development of remedial coping strategies.

Table 9.35 Psychosocial Concerns of HSCT Survivors

Physical Problems/ Medical Concerns	Psychological Problems	Community Reintegration Problems
• Fatigue • Treatment-related deconditioning • Appearance changes • Continued health problems • Cognitive impairment • Eating and sleeping problems • Physical restrictions • Sexual dysfunction, infertility • Immunosuppression, vulnerability to infections	• Fear about future (impact of illness on life span, finances, family, work, academic goals) • Loss of control/dependence on others • Feeling more cautious, hypervigilance regarding physical symptoms • Isolation, separation from family and social network • Fear of relapse, fear of death • Fear of delayed treatment related side effects (graft vs. host disease, cataracts, organ damage, secondary malignancies) • Guilt (survivor guilt, family burden, perception of diminished contribution to family and society) • Anger • Diminished self-worth (as damaged by treatment)	• Return to former roles (parenting, spousal, work, community) • Resumption of social relations (rejection sensitivity, social withdrawal) • Stigmatization, employment and insurance discrimination • Relationship problems • Financial insecurity (treatment related expenses/debt, reduced earning potential)

Lung Cancer

Lung cancer carries a heavy emotional burden because smoking contributes to the cancer in 87% cases. That means that patients feel guilt, responsibility, and the stigma of having caused their illness. As they are treated, they are faced with the challenge of trying to stop smoking or the guilt about continuing to smoke. While the 5-year survival of the patient with an isolated lung nodule is good, 60 percent of patients present with the grave prognosis of metastatic disease. Prognosis is directly related to quality of life and performance status. Patients fear the compromise of hypoxia, chronic coughing, and brain metastases.

Table 9.36 Treatments for Depression, Anxiety, and Nicotine Dependency

Depression
- At three months, rates of depression are 16 - 22%
- Small cell carcinoma in lung patients presents with more systemic malaise at the outset that can be treated by chemotherapy.
- Sense of effort and hopelessness may be mistaken for the limitations of post-surgical loss of fitness and the demands of more shortness of breath.
- Greater sense of effort or trouble in getting going
- Patients sigh more.
- Depression is usually more common among women.
- Men with lung cancer have a higher rate of depression when performance status is compromised. Physical limitations will mean that they must adjust to physical job disability. Loss of voice and lung power can mean loss of unique control and manhood.
- In the setting of nicotine withdrawal, depression and irritability are also more likely.
- Pain is worse with depression, and neuralgic pain post-thoracotomy may be amplified if the patient is depressed.
- Fatigue is one feature of depression.
  - Sleep disorder is common.
  - Lung radiation is associated with fatigue in most patients by the third week; about half are better at three months.
  - Postural hypotension related to chemotherapy can contribute to fatigue.
- Cf. Chapter 6, Mood Disorders.

- Antidepressants: *sertraline* (Zoloft®); *paroxetine* (Paxil®); *escitalopram* (Lexapro®); *fluoxetine* (Prozac®); *citalopram* (Celexa®); *venlafaxine* (Effexor®)
- Anxiolytics: *lorazepam* (Ativan®); *alprazolam* (Xanax®); *clonazepam* (Klonopin®)
- Psychotherapy
- Social support moderates the loss of physical function
- Treat pain.
- Lowering routine antihypertensive medications in the anti-cancer setting and attention to anemia may be helpful.
- SSRIs like *fluoxitene* (Prozac®) are also good for postural hypotension of autonomic dysfunction.
- Pulmonary rehabilitation and physical therapy are keys for increased stamina.

Anxiety
- Symptoms of a panic attack overlap with symptoms of lung and heart disease and fear of recurrent cancer.
- Symptoms are palpitations or tachycardia, shortness of breath, chest pain, nausea or abdominal distress, sweating, trembling and shaking, feeling of choking, dizziness or faintness, paresthesias, chills or hot flashes, derealization and depersonalization, fear of losing control or going crazy, and fear of dying.

- Benzodiazapines (anxiolytics): *lorazepam* (Ativan®); *alprazolam* (Xanax®)
- Antidepressants for chronic anxiety or recurrent panic attacks: SSRIs not sedating, no risk of contributing to respiratory depression, better to reduce the threshold to panic attacks than benzodiazapines as needed.

(continued, next page)

Table 9.36 Treatments for Depression, Anxiety, and Nicotine Dependency (continued)

Anxiety (continued)
- Pulmonary embolus can present with anxiety.
- A phobia of needles can complicate care in patients who must inject anticoagulant medications daily.

- Differential diagnosis of anxiety should include pulmonary embolus.
- Behavioral interventions (cf. Chapter 5)

Smoking cessation (cf. Head and Neck Cancer, Table 9.28)

- *Buproprion* (Wellbutrin®): antidepressant with record for reducing craving for cigarettes as well as improving mood; marketed for smoking cessation separately from Wellbutrin® as Zyban®; 150 mg bid in the slow release form; works best with counseling and cognitive behavioral treatments
- *Nortriptyline* (Pamelor®) has also been used in smoking cessation.
- Nicotine can be tapered via a variety of nicotine delivery systems.

Table 9.37 Treatments for Problems with Cognition*

Chronic hypoxia is a common reason for cognitive impairment

- Nighttime oxygen and daytime oxygen. The cognitive benefit of oxygen treatment is balanced against the embarrassment of carrying oxygen and appearing disabled.

Medications

- Eliminate benzodiazepines and anticholinergic medications

Brain metastases occur in 10-15% non-small cell cancer patients at presentation. They often develop early in the course of treatment for stage III disease. Risk of brain recurrence in small cell carcinoma within two years without prophylactic cranial radiation is 60-80%.

- For curable small cell lung cancer, protocols include prophylactic cranial irradiation.

Hypercalcemia and *hyponatremia* may contribute to delirium

- Correct calcium, sodium, magnesium.

* *Cf. Chapter 6, Cognitive Disorders.*

(continued, next page)

Table 9.37 Treatments for Problems with Cognition (continued)*

Cognitive impairment- common at diagnosis in these patients who are often *older smokers with vascular disease as well*

- Consider oxygen treatment at night or all day if chronically hypoxic.
- Check thyroid function tests, especially if radiation has been given near the neck in the past.

More rarely, cognition is impaired by *paraneoplastic effects* of the tumor. In these syndromes:
- low sodium occurs in 15%;
- ectopic adrenocorticotropic hormone produces Cushing's in 3%; and
- a paraneoplastic autoimmune encephalomyelitis, subacute sensory neuropathy, or temporo-limbic disease can occur rarely.

- Psychotropic medications may be useful to treat symptoms like psychosis, seizure, mood lability.

Limbic encephalitis is a rare syndrome associated with short-term memory deficits, seizures, and dementia.

- MRI can document this syndrome in 70% patients.
- Treatment of the tumor
- Ad hoc treatments with tranquilizers, anticonvulsants or antidepressants

Protocols have been adjusted to minimize *Leukoencephalopathy* - a structural change in cerebral white matter in which myelin suffers the most damage; the cognitive and emotional loss may be confused with clinical depression.
- Inattention, memory loss, and emotional dysfunction may be features of mild diffuse white matter damage.
- More severe cases present as dementia, abulia, stupor, or coma.
- Language ability and praxis are often preserved.
- Abnormality on brain MRI documents the diagnosis.
- Sometimes decreased density of white matter can be noted on brain CT.

- Neuropsychological testing
- For syndromes of inattention, stimulants may have a role, e.g. *modafinil* (Provigil®) and *methylphenidate* (Ritalin®).

* Cf. Chapter 6, Cognitive Disorders.

Table 9.38 Side Effects of Chemotherapy that Affect Mental Status*

Medication	Symptom and Treatment
Ifosfamide	Transient delirium and ataxia mid treatment
Etoposide	Postural hypotension
Cisplatin	Leukoencephalopathy and peripheral neuropathy
Dexamethasone (Decadron®) and *prednisone* (Deltasone®) • Commonly used for lung disease and brain or spinal cord metastases. • Risk is dose related. • Prednisone 60 mg is equivalent to 9 mg dexamethasone.	• Cause mood instability, insomnia, jitteriness, increased appetite, lability, tearfulness, hypomania, and irritability • Sometimes the mood crashes after steroids are decreased. • Stopping steroid medication does not always lead to rapid improvement; psychotropic interventions are typically necessary. • Effective treatments are antipsychotic medications, mood stabilizers, and *carbamzepine* (Tegretol®). Phenothiazines, *haloperidol* (Haldol®), *olanzapine* (Zyprexa®), and *risperidone* (Risperdal®) are helpful in the acute setting.

* *Cf. Chapter 6, Cognitive Disorders.*

Melanoma

For high-risk melanoma, surveillance is every 3-4 months for 2 years, then every 6 months for 3 years for high-risk melanoma. For low risk melanoma, NCCN recommends visits every 6 months for 2 years then annually. Melanoma is known for its variable course and its sensitivity to immunological treatments. It is also notable for its high rate of recurrence in the central nervous system. The main source of anxiety is the worry about recurrence. We know from major studies that psychosocial interventions effectively ease the distress related to this diagnosis.

Table 9.39 Interventions for Side Effects of Melanoma Treatments*

Interferon-alpha - *prescribed for as long as a year at moderate doses to reduce the risk of recurrence in patients with advanced melanoma*

• Anxiety, insomnia, a motor restlessness or akathisia • Clinical depression, suicidal thoughts. Symptoms of depression can include irritability, insomnia, excessive guilt, and tearfulness, difficulties with concentration and clarity of thought. • Occasionally hypomania, mania or psychosis	• Antidepressant medication is effective for the major depressive disorder caused by interferon-alpha. Serotonin reuptake inhibitors are used most commonly. • In order to reduce risk of depression, antidepressants may be started three weeks in advance. • Consider autoimmune thyroiditis as a cause of anxiety or fatigue and depression. Patients may have transient hyperthyroidism or hypothyroidism. Monitor thyroid function. • Interferon-alpha can inhibit P450 isoenzymes CYP1A2, 2D6 and 2C19, delaying metabolism of some antidepressants. Higher doses of antidepressant may lead to higher serum levels and side effects. • If an antidepressant medication is not working, reconsider the diagnosis. The patient may be manic, hypomanic, hypothyroid, or suffering side effects of the antidepressant. • Benzodiazepines for anxiety, antidepressant medications for interferon-alpha- induced depression, mood stabilizers for mood lability or hypomania.
• Flu-like syndrome with the fever, body aches, malaise and fatigue normally associated with a viral condition.	• Acetaminophen for flu-like syndrome
• Occasionally, severe psychiatric side effects: confusion, suicidal thoughts, and hallucinations	• Typically clear with cessation of cancer treatment

Interleukin-2 (IL-2)

• Flu syndrome, depressive symptoms, and confusion as part of a capillary leak syndrome; impairments of working spatial memory and planning have been noted after 5 days; pattern differs some from the psychiatric side effects of interferon-alpha alone.	• Resolve after treatment.

* Cf. Chapter 6, Anxiety, Mood Disorders.

Table 9.40 Interventions for Psychological Issues with Melanoma

Management of risk for other fair-skinned, redheaded, or high-risk family members with family history melanoma, dysplastic nevi	• Hear the patient out. • Consider genetic counseling. • Educate family members about risk.
Guilt about sun exposure and risk taking	• Help patient focus on present, not past. • Screening by regular dermatological evaluation.
Anxiety due to risk of recurrence	• Psychosocial interventions to cope with anxiety (cf. Chapter 6, Anxiety) • Cognitive-behavioral therapy (cf. Chapter 5) • Education about melanoma • Relaxation techniques (cf. Chapter 5) • Group and individual interventions • Educate patient about variable course of disease.
High risk of central nervous system metastases, often hemorrhagic.	• Hear out concerns about changes in neurological function and carefully assess medically.

References

Brain Cancer

1. Valentine AD, Passik SD & Massie MJ (2005). Psychiatric and psychosocial issues. In VA Levin (Ed.), *Cancer in the nervous system* (pp. 572-579). New York: Oxford University Press.

2. National Cancer Institute (NCI). (2004). *SEER Cancer Statistics Review, 1975-2001.* Bethesda, MD: Author.

3. Central Brain Tumor Registry of the United States (CBTRUS). (2002). *Statistical Report: Primary Brain Tumors in the United States, 1995-1999.* Hinsdale, IL: Author.

4. Yung WK, Kunschner LJ, Sawaya R, Chang CL & Fuller GM (2002). Intracranial Metastases. In VA Levin (Ed.), *Cancer in the nervous system* (pp.321-340). New York: Oxford University Press.

5. Delattre JY, Krol G, Thaler HT & Posner JB (1988). Distribution of brain metastases. *Archives of Neurology, 45,* 741-744.

6. Grossman SA & Krabak MJ (1999). Leptomeningeal carcinomatosis. *Cancer Treatment Reviews, 25,* 103-119.

7. Meyers CA & Kayl AE (2002). Neurocognitive dysfunction. In VA Levin (Ed.), *Cancer in the nervous system* (pp. 557-571). New York: Oxford University Press.

8. Duffy JD & Campbell JJ (1994). The regional prefrontal syndromes: A theoretical and clinical overview. *The Journal of Neuropsychiatry and Clinical Neurosciences, 6,* 379-3987.

9. Wellisch DK, Kaleita TA, Freeman D, Cloughesy T & Goldman J (2002). Predicting major depression in brain tumor patients. *Psycho-Oncology, 11,* 230-238.

10. Litofsky NS, Farace E, Anderson F, Meyers CA, Huang W, Laws ER, et al. (2004). Depression in patients with high-grade glioma: Results of the Glioma Outcomes Project. *Neurosurgery, 54,* 358-366.

11. New P (2001). Radiation injury to the nervous system. *Current Opinion in Neurology, 14,* 725-734.

12. Keime-Guibert F, Napolitano M & Delattre JY (1998). Neurological complications of radiotherapy and chemotherapy. *Journal of Neurology, 245,* 695-708.

13. Warren KE & Fine HA (2002). Systemic chemotherapy of central nervous system tumors. In M Prados (Ed.), *American cancer society atlas of clinical oncology: Brain cancer* (pp. 193-210). Hamilton, Ontario: BC Decker, Inc.

14. Meyers CA, Weitzner MA, Valentine AD & Levin VA (1998). Methylphenidate therapy improves cognition, mood, and function of brain tumor patients. *Journal of Clinical Oncology, 16,* 2522-2527.

Breast Cancer

15. Rowland JH & Massie MJ (2004). Issues in breast cancer survivorship. In JR Harris, ME Lippman, M Morrow & CK Osbourne (Eds.), *Diseases of the breast* (3rd ed. pp. 1419-1452). Lippincott, PA: Williams and Wilkins.

16. Massie MJ & Greenberg D (2004). Oncology. In J Levenson, (Ed.), *APPI textbook of psychosomatic medicine* (pp.597-618). Washington, DC: American Psychiatric Press.

17. Robson ME & Offit K (2002). Considerations in genetic counseling for inherited breast cancer predisposition. *Seminars in Radiation Oncology, 12,* 362-370.

18. Robson ME, Boyd J, Borgen PI & Cody HS (2001). Hereditary breast cancer. *Current Problems in Surgery, 38,* 377-480.

19. Stearns V, Isaacs C, Rowland J, Crawford J, Ellis MJ, Kramer R, et al. (2000). A pilot trial assessing the efficacy of paroxetine hydrochloride (Paxil) in controlling hot flashes in breast cancer survivors. *Annals of Oncology*, *11*, 17-22.

20. Duffy LS, Greenberg DB, Younger J & Ferraro MG (1999). Iatrogenic acute estrogen deficiency and psychiatric syndromes in breast cancer patients. *Psychosomatics*, *40*, 304-308.

21. American Cancer Society, Treatment Topics & Resources, Staying Active During Treatment, Sexuality for Women and Their Partners. Retrieved 21 February 2006 at http://www.cancer.org/docroot/MIT/MIT_7_1x_SexualityforWomenandTheir Partners.asp?.

Gastrointestinal Cancer

22. Gelfand GA & Finley RJ (1994). Quality of life with carcinoma of the esophagus. *World Journal of Surgical Oncology*, *18*, 399-405.

23. Padilla GV, Grant MM, Lipsett J, Anderson PR, Rhiner M & Bogen C (1992). Health quality of life and colorectal cancer. *Cancer*, *70*, 1450-1456.

24. Wade BE (1990). Colostomy patients: Psychological adjustment at 10 weeks and 1 year after surgery in districts which employed stoma-care nurses and districts which did not. *Journal of Advanced Nursing*, *15*, 1297-1304.

25. Sprangers MAG, Taal BG, Aaronson NK & te Velde A (1995). Quality of life in colorectal cancer. Stoma vs. nonstoma patients. *Diseases of the Colon and Rectum*, *38*, 361-369.

26. Barsevick AM, Pasacreta J & Orsi A (1995). Psychological distress and functional dependency in colorectal cancer patients. *Cancer Practice*, *3*, 105-110.

27. Nordin K & Glimelius B (1997). Psychological reactions in newly diagnosed gastrointestinal cancer patients. *Acta Oncologica*, *36*, 803-810.

28. Ebrahimi B, Tucker SL, Li D, Abbruzzese JL & Kurzrock R (2004). Cytokines in pancreatic carcinoma. *Cancer*, *101*, 2727-2736.

29. Musselman DL, Miller AH, Porter MR, Manatunga A, Gao F, Penna S, et al. (2001). Higher than normal interleukin-6 concentrations in cancer patients with depression: Preliminary findings. *The American Journal of Psychiatry*, *158*, 1252-1257.

30. Musselman DL, Lawson DH, Gumnick JF, Manatunga AK, Penna S, Goodkin RS, et al. (2001). Paroxetine for the prevention of depression induced by high-dose interferon alfa. *New England Journal of Medicine*, *344*, 961-966.

Genitourinary Cancer

31. Barton D & Loprinzi CL (2004). Making sense of the evidence regarding nonhormonal treatments for hot flashes. *Clinical Journal of Oncology Nursing, 8,* 39-42.

32. Eton DT & Lepore SJ (2002). Prostate cancer and health-related quality of life: A review of the literature. *Psycho-Oncology, 11,* 307-326.

33. Fossa SD, Dahl AA & Loge JH (2003). Fatigue, anxiety, and depression in long-term survivors of testicular cancer. *Journal of Clinical Oncology, 21,* 1249-1254.

34. Kornblith AB, Herr HW, Ofman US, Scher HI & Holland JC (1994). Quality of life of patients with prostate cancer and their spouses. The value of a database in clinical care. *Cancer, 73,* 2791-2802.

35. Litwin MS, Lubeck DP, Henning JM & Carroll PR (1998). Differences in urologist and patient assessments of health related quality of life in men with prostate cancer: Results of the CaPSURE database. *The Journal of Urology, 159,*1988-1992.

36. Nelson CJ, Rosenfeld S & Roth AJ (2005). Coping with your diagnosis and moving forward. In DG Bostwick, ED Crawford, CS Higano, M Roach (Eds.). *American Cancer Society Health Promotions, American Cancer Society's complete guide to prostate cancer* (pp.81-88). Atlanta, GA: ACS.

37. Palapattu GS, Haisfield-Wolfe ME, Walker JM, BrintzenhofeSzoc K, Trock B, Zabora J, et al. (2004). Assessment of perioperative psychological distress in patients undergoing radical cystectomy for bladder cancer. *J Urol., 172* (5 Pt 1), 1814-1817.

38. Penson DF & Litwin MS (2003). Quality of life after treatment for prostate cancer. *Current Urology Reports, 4,* 185-195.

39. Pirl WF, Siegel GI, Goode MJ & Smith MR (2002). Depression in men receiving androgen deprivation therapy for prostate cancer: A pilot study. *Psycho-Oncology, 11,* 518-523.

40. Roth AJ, Kornblith AB, Batel-Copel L, Peabody E, Scher HI & Holland JC (1998). Rapid screening for psychologic distress in men with prostate carcinoma: A pilot study. *Cancer, 82,* 1904-1908.

41. Roth AJ, Rosenfeld B, Kornblith AB, Gibson C, Scher HI, Curley-Smart T, et al. (2003) The memorial anxiety scale for prostate cancer: Validation of a new scale to measure anxiety in men with prostate cancer. *Cancer, 97,* 2910-2918.

42. Schover LR (1997). *Sexuality and fertility after cancer.* New York: Wiley.

Gynecological Cancer

43. Auchincloss SS & McCartney CF (1998). Gynecologic cancer. In R McCorkle (Ed.), *Psychological issues related to site of cancer*. In: Holland, J.C. Psycho-oncology. New York: Oxford Press 359-370.

44. Epocrates mobile drug and formulary reference. (2005). Pharmacological data retrieved 19 December 2005 from http://www2.epocrates.com/index.html.

45. Moore S (2004). Menopausal symptoms. In CH Yarbro, M Goodman &MH Frogge (Eds.), *Cancer symptom management* (3rd ed., pp.571-595). Boston, MA: Jones and Bartlett Publishers.

46. Bruner DW & Berk L (2004). Altered body image and sexual health. In CH Yarbro, M Goodman & MH Frogge (Eds.), *Cancer symptom management* (3rd ed., pp.596-632). Boston, MA: Jones and Bartlett Publishers.

47. Schover LR (1997). *Sexuality and fertility after cancer*. New York: Wiley.

48. Schover LR (1998). Sexual dysfunction. In W Breitbart (Ed.), Management of specific symptoms. In JC Holland (Ed.), *Psycho-oncology*. New York: Oxford Press 494-499. Epocrates 2005.

Head and Neck Cancer

49. Espie CA, Freedlander E, Campsie LM, Soutar DS & Robertson AG (1989). Psychological distress at follow-up after major surgery for intra-oral cancer. *Journal of Psychosomatic Research*, 33, 441-448.

50. Ackerstaff AH, Hilgers FJM, Aaronson NK & Balm AJM (1994). Communication, functional disorders and lifestyle changes after total laryngectomy. *Clinical Otolaryngology*, 19, 295-300

51. List MA, Stracks J, Colangelo L, Butler P, Ganzenko N, Lundy D, et al. (2000). How do head and neck cancer patients prioritize treatment outcomes before initiating treatment? *Journal of Clinical Oncology*, 18, 877-884.

52. List MA, Siston A, Haraf D, Schumm P, Kies M, Stenson K, et al. (1999). Quality of life and performance in advanced head and neck cancer patients on concomitant chemoradiotherapy: A prospective examination. *Journal of Clinical Oncology*, 17,1020-1028.

53. Hammerlid E, Bjordal K, Ahlner-Elmqvist M, Boysen M, Evensen JF, Biorklund A, et al. (2001). A prospective study of quality of life in head and neck cancer patients. Part I: At diagnosis. *The Laryngoscope*, 111, 669-680.

54. de Graeff A, Leeuw JR, Ros WJ, Hordijk GJ, Blijham & Winnubst JA (1999). A prospective study on quality of life of patients with cancer of the oral cavity or oropharynx treated with surgery with or without radiotherapy. *Oral Oncology, 35*, 27-32.

55. Weymuller EA, Alsarraf R, Yueh B, Deleyiannis FWB & Coltrera MD (2001). Analysis of the performance characteristics of the University of Washington quality of life instrument and its modification (UW-QOL-R). *Archives of Otolaryngolology – Head and Neck Surgery, 127*, 489-493.

56. List MA, D'Antonio LL, Cella DF, Siston A, Mumby P, Haraf D, et al. (1996). The performance status scale for head and neck cancer patients and the functional assessment of cancer therapy-head and neck scale. A study of utility and validity. *Cancer, 77*, 2294-2301.

Hematological Cancer

57. Andrykowski MA, Bishop MM, Hahn EA, Cella DF, Beaumont JL, Brady MJ, et al. (2005). Long-term health related quality of life and spiritual well-being after hematopoietic stem cell transplantation. *Journal of Clinical Oncology, 23*, 599-608.

58. Andrykowski MA & McQuellon RP (1998). Bone marrow transplantation. In R McCorkle (Ed.), Psychological responses to treatment. In JC Holland (Ed.), *Psycho-oncology* (pp.289-299). New York: Oxford University Press.

59. Bellm LA, Epstein JB, Rose-Ped A, Martin P & Fuchs HJ (2000). Patient reports of complications of bone marrow transplantation. *Support Care Cancer, 8*, 33-39.

60. Fann JR, Roth-Roemer S, Burington BE, Katon WJ & Syrjala KL (2002). Delirium in patients undergoing hematopoietic stem cell transplantation. *Cancer, 95*, 1971-1981.

61. Fann JR, Alfano CM, Burington BE, Roth-Roemer S, Katon WJ & Syrjala KL (2005). Clinical presentation of delirium in patients undergoing hematopoietic stem cell transplantation. Delirium and distress symptoms and time course. *Cancer, 103*, 810-820.

62. Harder H, Cornelissen JJ, Van Gool AR, Duivenvoorden HJ, Eijkenbook WM & van den Bent MJ (2002). Cognitive functioning and quality of life in long term survivors of bone marrow transplantation. *Cancer, 95*, 183-192.

63. Lesko LM (1998). Hematopoietic dyscrasias. In R McCorkle (Ed.), Psychological issues related to site of cancer. In JC Holland (Ed.), *Psycho-Oncology* (pp.406-416). New York: Oxford University Press.

64. Roth AG & Holland JC (2003) Psychological aspects of hematological malignancies. In PH Wiernik, JM Goldman, JP Dutcher & RA Kyle (Eds.), *Neoplastic diseases of the blood* (4th ed.) (pp. 1155-1165). New York: Cambridge University Press.

65. Syrjala KL, Dikmen S, Langer SL, Roth-Roemer S, Abrams JR (2004). Neuropsychologic changes from before transplantation to 1 year in patients receiving myeloablative allogeneic hematopoietic cell transplant. *Blood, 104*, 3386-3392.

Lung Cancer

66. Darnell RB & Posner JB (2003). Paraneoplastic syndromes involving the nervous system. *New England Journal of Medicine, 349*, 1543-1554.

67. Filley CM & Kleinschmidt-DeMasters BK (2001). Toxic leukoencephalopathy. *New England Journal of Medicine, 345*, 425-432.

68. Hopwood P & Stephens RJ (2000). Depression in patients with lung cancer: Prevalence and risk factors derived from quality-of-life data. *Journal of Clinical Oncology, 18*, 893-903.

69. King KB, Nail LM, Kreamer K. Strohl RA & Johnson JE (1985). Patients' descriptions of the experience of receiving radiation therapy. *Oncology Nursing Forum, 12*, 55-61.

70. Nocturnal Oxygen Therapy Trial Group (NOTTG). (1980). Continuous or nocturnal oxygen therapy in hypoxemic chronic obstructive lung disease. *Annals of Internal Medicine, 93*, 391-398.

71. Stuschke M, Eberhardt W, Pottgen C, Stamatis G, Wilke H, Stoblen G, et al. (1999). Prophylactic cranial irradiation in locally advanced non-small-cell lung cancer after multimodality treatment: Long-term follow-up and investigations of late neuropsychologic effects. *Journal of Clinical Oncology, 17*, 2700-2709.

72. The Tobacco Use and Dependence Clinical Practice Guideline Panel, Staff, and Consortium Representatives. (2000). A clinical practice guideline for treating tobacco use and dependence. A US Public Health Service Report. *The Journal of the American Medical Association, 283*, 3244-3254.

73. Uchitomi Y, Mikami I, Kugaya A, Akizuki N, Nagai K, Nishiwaki Y, et al. (2000). Depression after successful treatment for nonsmall cell lung carcinoma: A 3-month follow-up study. *Cancer, 89*, 1172-1179.

74. Zabora J, BrintzenhofeSzoc K, Curbow B, Hooker C & Piantadosi S (2001). The prevalence of psychological distress by cancer site. *Psycho-Oncology, 10*, 19-28.

Melanoma

75. Boesen EH, Ross L, Frederiksen K, Thomsen BL, Dahlstrom K, Schmidt G, et al. (2005). Psychoeducational intervention for patients with cutaneous malignant melanoma: A replication study. *Journal of Clinical Oncology*, 23, 1270-1277.

76. Bunston T, Mackie A, Jones D & Mings D (1994). Identifying the nonmedical concerns of patients with ocular melanoma. *Journal of Opthalmic Nursing & Technology*, 13, 227-237.

77. Capuron L, Ravaud A & Dantzer R (2000). Early depressive symptoms in cancer patients receiving interleukin-2 and/or interferon alfa-2b therapy. *Journal of Clinical Oncology*, 18, 2143-2151.

78. Caraceni A, Gangeri L, Martini C, Belli F, Brunelli C, Baldini M, et al. (1998). Neurotoxicity of interferon alpha in melanoma therapy: Results from a randomized controlled trial. *Cancer*, 83, 482-489.

79. Fawzy FI, Canada AL, Fawzy NW (2003). Effects of a brief, structured psychiatric intervention on survival and recurrence at 10-year follow-up. *Archives of General Psychiatry*, 60, 100-103.

80. Fawzy FI, Cousins N, Fawzy NW, Kemeny ME, Elashoff R & Morton D (1990). A structured psychiatric intervention for cancer patients: I. Changes over time in methods of coping and affective disturbance. *Archives of General Psychiatry*, 47, 720-725.

81. Fawzy FI, Kemeny ME, Fawzy N, Elashoff R, Morton D, Cousins M, et al. (1990). A structured psychiatric intervention for cancer patients: II. Changes over time in immunological measures. *Archives of General Psychiatry*, 47, 729-735.

82. Fawzy FI, Fawzy NW, Hyun CS, Elashoff R, Guthrie D, Fahey JL, et al. (1993). Malignant melanoma. Effects of an early structured psychiatric intervention, coping, and affective state on recurrence and survival 6 years later. *Archives of General Psychiatry*, 50, 681-689.

83. Kirkwood JM, Bender C, Agarwala S, Tarhini A, Shipe-Spotloe J, Smelko B, et al. (2002). Mechanisms and management of toxicities associated with high-dose interferon alfa-2b therapy. *Journal of Clinical Oncology*, 20, 3703-3718.

84. Musselman DL, Lawson DH, Gumnick JF, Manatunga AK, Penna S, Goodkin RS, et al. (2001). Paroxetine for the prevention of depression induced by high-dose interferon alfa. *New England Journal of Medicine*, 344, 961-966.

85. Sher D, Greenberg D, Ebb DH, Mazzoni P & Pirl W (2004). Clinical implications of psychosis during interferon treatment for giant cell tumor. [Abstract] P8-2. *Psycho-oncology*, 13 S40.

General Cancer Information

The National Cancer Institute
www.nci.org
The NCI conducts and supports research, training, health information dissemination, and other programs with respect to the cause, diagnosis, prevention, and treatment of cancer, rehabilitation from cancer, and the continuing care of cancer patients and the families of cancer patients.

American Cancer Society
http://www.cancer.org/docroot/home/index.asp
The American Cancer Society is the nationwide community- based voluntary health organization dedicated to eliminating cancer as a major health problem by preventing cancer, saving lives, and diminishing suffering from cancer, through research, education, advocacy, and service.

American Society of Clinical Oncology
http://www.asco.org
The American Society of Clinical Oncology (ASCO) is the world's leading professional organization representing physicians who treat people with cancer through more effective treatments, increased funding for clinical and translational research, and cures.

American College of Surgeons
http://www.facs.org
The American College of Surgeons is a scientific and educational association dedicated to improving the care of the surgical patient and to safeguarding standards of care in an optimal and ethical practice environment.

American Society for Therapeutic Radiology and Oncology (ASTRO)
http://www.astro.org
ASTRO is dedicated to improving patient care through education, the advancement of science and representing radiation oncology in the health policy arena.

(continued, next page)

American Psychosocial Oncology Society (APOS)
http://www.apos-society.org
APOS includes all health care professionals who seek to advance the science and practice of psychosocial care for people with cancer.

International Psycho-Oncology Society (IPOS)
http://www.ipos-society.org
IPOS is the international, multidisciplinary organization dedicated to the science of psychosocial and behavioral oncology and improving the care of cancer patients and their families throughout the world.

Patient Education, Information, Advocacy and Support

American Psychosocial Oncology Society *Helpline*
http://www.apos-society.org/survivors/helpline
APOS *Helpline* is a toll-free hot line (1-866-276-7443 or 1-866-APOS-4-HELP) for cancer patients and advocacy organizations to obtain referrals for local counseling and support services throughout the United States.

Cancer Care
http://www.cancercare.org/
Cancer*Care* is a national non-profit organization whose mission is to provide free professional help to people with all cancers through counseling, education, information and referral and direct financial assistance.

Lance Armstrong Foundation (LAF)
http://www.laf.org/
 LAF provides practical information and tools for people living with cancer through four core program areas: Education, Advocacy, Public Health and Research.

The National Coalition of Cancer Survivorship
www.canceradvocacy.org/
The National Coalition for Cancer Survivorship is the oldest survivor-led advocacy organization working on behalf of people with all types of cancer and their families.

National Patient Advocate Association
http://www.npaf.org/
National Patient Advocate Foundation seeks to create avenues of access to insurance funding for evolving therapies, therapeutic devices and agents through legislative and policy reform.

OncoLink
http://www.oncolink.com/
OncoLink was founded in 1994 by The University of Pennsylvania's cancer specialists with a mission to help cancer patients, families, health care professionals and the general public get accurate cancer-related information at no charge.

People Living With Cancer
www.plwc.org
People Living With Cancer, the patient information website of the American Society of Clinical Oncology (ASCO), provides oncologist-approved information on more than 50 types of cancer and their treatments, clinical trials, coping, and side effects.

The Wellness Community
www.thewellnesscommunity.org
The Wellness Community (TWC) is an international non-profit organization dedicated to providing free emotional support, education and hope for people with cancer and their loved ones.

Caregiver Resources

The National Family Caregivers Association
http://www.nfcacares.org/
The National Family Caregivers Association (NFCA) supports, empowers, educates, and speaks up for the more than 50 million Americans who care for a chronically ill, aged, or disabled loved one.

Children and Families

The National Childhood Cancer Foundation
www.curesearch.org
On this site you will find information which addresses all aspects of the care of children with cancer.. On

Childrens Oncology Group
www.childrensoncologygroup.org
The mission of the Childrens Oncology Group is cure and prevent childhood and adolescent cancer through scientific discovery and compassionate care.

Bereavement and Grief Counseling

Association for Death Education and Counseling
http://www.adec.org
ADEC is dedicated to promoting excellence in death education, care of the dying, and bereavement counseling through its multicultural and multidisciplinary membership.

The American Academy of Hospice and Palliative Medicine (AAHPM)
http://www.aahpm.org
AAHPM is dedicated to the advancement of palliative medicine through prevention and relief of patient and family suffering by providing education and clinical practice standards, fostering research, facilitating personal and professional development, and by public policy advocacy.

Index

A

acetaminophen (Tylenol®)
    for pain, 80, 83
activity level
    and fatigue, 75
acute confusional state, 51
acute lymphoblastic leukemia (ALL), 140
acute myeloid leukemia (AML), 140
acute radiation syndrome, 110
addiction, 58
adjustment disorders, 45
adolescents
    developmental guidelines, 45
aggressive lymphomas, 144
agitation
    algorithm for medicating, 22
    differential diagnosis, 21
    reducing in patient, 21
akathisia, 41
albuterol inhaler, 41
alchohol withdrawal, 136
    treatment strategies, 135
alemtuzumab
    vomiting risk, 87
alibido, 92
alpha agonists
    for delirium, 54
alprazolam (Xanax®), 30
    for anti-estrogen side effect, 117
    for anxiety, 42, 43
    for brain tumor, 112
    for breast cancer, 115
    for depression with lung cancer, 148
    for genitourinary cancer, 124
    for gynecological cancer anxiety, 130

in psychiatric emergency, 20
    for smoking cessation, 135
aluminum hydroxide
    for mouth pain, 137
American Academy of Hospice and
        Palliative Medicine, 164
American Brain Tumor Foundation, 112
American Cancer Society, 161
American College of Surgeons, 161
American Psychosocial Oncology Society
        (APOS), 162
    Helpline, 37, 162
American Society for Therapeutic
        Radiology and Oncology, 161
American Society of Clinical Oncology, 161
amifostine
    vomiting risk, 87
amitriptyline (Elavil®), 29, 50
    for breast cancer, 116
    for neuropathic pain, 83
d-amphetamine, 50
    for brain tumor, 112
anemia
    and fatigue, 74
anesthetics
    for delirium, 54
angry patient, 66
anhedonia, 45
Annon's PLISSIT Model of sexual
        assessment, 90
anticipatory nausea, 86
    behavioral management, 90
antidepressants, 26, 27, 49, 50
    for anxiety, 43
    for brain cancer, 112

for breast cancer, 116
tricyclics, 29
anti-estrogens
psychiatric side effects, 117
antipsychotic drugs, 31, 43, 50
for delirium, 53
in psychiatric emergency, 20
antisocial personality disorder, 62
anxiety
brain tumor and, 110
coping techniques, 33
disorders, 39-44
drug management, 43
etiology, 40-41
evaluation, 42
gynecological cancer and, 130
interventions, 42
lung cancer and, 148-149
and pain, 79
psychotherapy and behavioral
interventions, 44
signs and symptoms, 39, 40
vs. substance abuse, 58
anxiolytics
for brain tumor, 112
apathetic syndrome, 109
aprepitant (Emend®)
arousal, 91
arsenic trioxide
vomiting risk, 87
art therapy, 37
L-asparaginase
and depression, 47
vomiting risk, 87
Association for Death Education and
Counseling, 164
attention
reduced ability to maintain, 14
avoidant personality disorder, 62
awareness
Memorial Delirium Assessment Scale, 13

B
B-12
and depression, 46
barbiturates
and depression, 46
Beck Depression Inventory, 47
behavioral management
for fatigue treatment, 77
benzocaine (Orajel®)
for mouth pain, 137
benzodiazepines, 27
for anxiety, 43
for breast cancer, 116
for delirium, 53
and depression, 47
for genitourinary cancer, 124
for gynecological cancer anxiety, 130
for nausea and vomiting, 88
for pain treatment, 80
for smoking cessation, 135
in psychiatric emergency, 20
benztropine (Cogentin®), 41
for gynecological cancer, 130
bereavement counseling, 164
bexarotene
vomiting risk, 87
biofeedback, 34
in pain management, 85
bisphosphonates
for bone pain, 81
black cohosh
for premature menopause, 132
bladder cancer
preoperative chemotherapy, 127
psychosocial issues, 122
radical cystectomy, 126
bleomycin
vomiting risk, 87
bone pain, 81
borderline personality disorder, 58, 62

vomiting, 85-90
   behavioral management, 89
   radiation-induced, 88
   risk from chemotherapy agents, 87
   treatments, 88
vulvar atrophy, 132

W

Watson Scoring Method
   for mini mental status exam, 12
weight gain
   as anti-estrogen side effect, 117
weight loss
   in pancreatic cancer, 121
Wellness Community, 36, 163
"white coat syndrome", 41
wild yam
   for premature menopause, 132

X

xerostomia, 137

Z

zaleplon (Sonata®), 30
ziprasidone (Geodon®)
   for agitation, 22
   in psychiatric emergency, 20
zolpidem (Ambien®)
   for anti-estrogen side effect, 117
   for breast cancer, 116
   for gynecological cancer, 130
   for premature menopause, 132
zolpidem SR (Ambien CR®)
   for gynecological cancer, 130
Zung Depression Rating Scale
     (ZDRS), 8-9